STOP
OVEREATING
DURING
LOW BLOOD SUGARS
WITH DIABETES

Learn how to manage hypoglycemia with type 1 and type 2 diabetes...without eating everything in the kitchen.

by Ginger Vieira

Foreword by Mark Heyman, PhD, CDCES

For my BFF

Thank you for reminding me to check my blood sugar when we're having too much fun, for eating the glucose tab flavors I don't like, for learning everything you possibly can about diabetes, and for never judging my daily need for great (or cheap) chocolate.

Self-publishing takes a village.

This book is self-published, but that doesn't mean it was produced by one gal.

Here's a big thank you to the people who supported the production of this book:

Brent Burdick
Karl Richardson
Samantha Walsh
Tara Mayo
Neil Greathouse
Theresa Hastings
Mark Heyman

I truly appreciate your editing, ideas, more editing, and ongoing support!

Sincerely,
Ginger

Love the book?

Leave a 5-star review on Amazon!

RECOMMENDED READING:

- **Diabetes Sucks and You Can Handle It** by Mark Heyman, PhD
- **Exercise with Type 1 Diabetes** by Ginger Vieira
- **Emotional Eating with Diabetes** by Ginger Vieira
- **Dealing with Diabetes Burnout** by Ginger Vieira
- **Think Like a Pancreas** by Gary Scheiner, MS, CDCES
- **Thriving with Diabetes** by Paul Rosman, DO, & David Edelman
- **Type 1 Diabetes: One Day at a Time** by Neil Greathouse
- **Type One Determination** by Lauren Plunkett
- **Sugar Surfing** by Stephen Ponder, MD & Kevin L. McMahon
- **Brights Spots & Landmines** by Adam Brown
- **Balancing Diabetes** by Kerri Sparling
- **Pumping Insulin** by John Walsh and Ruth Roberts

TABLE OF CONTENTS

Foreword

by Mark Heyman, PhD, CDCES

Low blood sugar is no fun.

At the very least, a low blood sugar episode can bring on some uncomfortable symptoms that can wear you out, slow you down, and make you feel self-conscious.

And sometimes low blood sugar can be downright terrifying.

Over the past 25 years of living with type I diabetes, I've had my fair share of both uncomfortable and sometimes scary low blood sugars. I've also over-treated my lows more times than I'd like to admit.

Additionally, over the past 10 years in my work as a diabetes psychologist, I've seen the stress that low blood sugar puts on people living with this condition. Unfortunately, even with the advanced treatments for managing blood glucose, we have available to us, it's not possible to eliminate the possibility of low blood sugar. However, we can learn skills to manage low blood sugar safely and effectively, to make sure it has as little impact on our lives as possible.

I have found that diabetes education is the foundation for managing the emotional challenges of living with diabetes, which includes how we think about, react to, and treat low blood sugars. If you don't know why you are feeling a certain way when you are low, how to treat your lows, and what is causing your lows, your go-to strategy when you have a low blood sugar is to overtreat it.

And we all know that overtreating your lows is your ticket to getting on the blood sugar rollercoaster.

With honesty, simplicity, and a healthy dose of humor (and sass!), Ginger gives us a step-by-step process to follow to help us stop over-treating low blood sugar. The elegance of this book lies in both its simplicity and practicality. Ginger not only explains complex physiological and psychological concepts in a way that is simple and easy to understand, but she uses these concepts to demonstrate the tactical steps we need to take to stop (or significantly reduce the chances of) overtreating our lows.

What truly sets this book apart is its practical approach. Each chapter will not only teach you important information about what diabetes is but also give you practical tips for how to use this information to improve how you think about and manage those pesky low blood sugars. Ginger's insights and guidance are not just from a textbook — she does a fantastic job of using reliable examples from her own life to show how she has put these tools to work in her own life.

As you dive into the book, I encourage you to approach what you learn with an open mind. Changing how you think about — and react to — low blood sugars is no easy task, and at times, you may doubt your ability to do it. But trust me when I tell you that with practice, patience, and the tools in this book, you will surprise yourself and see real progress, both with your blood sugars and stress levels.

This book is truly a guide for anyone seeking to change their approach to managing low blood sugars so they can get off the blood sugar rollercoaster and start managing their glucose with intention. I hope that after reading this book, you'll have the knowledge, skills, and confidence you need to be able to deal with low blood sugar, but not let a low blood sugar episode ruin your day.

Welcome to the first day of changing your approach to low blood sugar!

Mark Heyman, PhD, CDCES
TheDiabetesPsychologist.com

Introduction

Every low blood sugar feels a little different — depending on what you're doing when it hits.

Maybe it starts with a quiet feeling in your brain. That feeling becomes a soft voice whispering "problem" over and over. Within a few minutes, the whispers of "problem" suddenly become whispers of "emergency."

Your face and your chest start heating up. Your fingers start to tremble. Your legs feel suddenly unreasonably weak. Your thoughts become jumbled. You can't think straight.

"Emergency. Emergency. Emergency." It's no longer a whisper. It's a voice shouting, but you're the only one who can hear it. Your blood sugar is dropping. Hypoglycemia has arrived.

Panic. Danger. Emergency.

The simplest way to save yourself is by eating carbohydrates.

Your brain is desperately begging you to eat more, more, more. Eat all the cereal. Drink the whole carton of juice. Eat everything that's left in that pint of ice cream. Have a few of those granola bars. All of the jelly beans. Whatever you can find. It's brutal. You're trying to stay alive, but even when you've had enough, your brain still begs for more.

Even when the trembling and the sweating stop, your brain still wants more. Your body still feels like it's suffering; food is the only thing that helps you feel safe.

The 50 mg/dL will eventually be 300 mg/dL. And you know it even while you're eating, but you don't want to stop. Every inch of your body still feels like it's in danger. So you keep eating until that emergency siren starts to quiet down. It takes so long. Too long.

This may sound dramatic, but it's true: the habit of binge eating during low blood sugars can wreak havoc on your entire life.

We can call it a few things:

- Binge eating during lows
- Overeating during lows
- Over-treating lows

Whatever you want to call it, it creates a vicious cycle fueled by panic that drains your energy, your self-esteem, and your ability to get through the day safely and comfortably. It can affect many parts of your health beyond your blood sugar levels.

This vicious cycle can feel impossible to break out of when you're taking insulin on a daily basis.

But it's just a habit. And you can change this habit. It's a habit that starts with several self-destructive beliefs about managing lows and your own behavior, followed by a lack of personal guidelines for treating lows.

In this book, you'll look first at those self-destructive beliefs and the vicious cycle behind overeating during lows. You'll acknowledge the things you're telling yourself that encourage this self-abusive binge-eating habit to continue. You'll get real about the impact it can have on your entire life and why it's not an inevitable part of living with diabetes and taking insulin.

Then, you'll learn how to build a totally new way of thinking about lows and managing the panic. You'll develop new beliefs and personalized guidelines to help you thoughtfully prevent and manage lows.

Chapter I

THE VICIOUS CYCLE OF OVERTREATING LOWS

The chaos that comes with the vicious cycle of overeating during low blood sugars wreaks havoc on far more than your blood sugars later that day.

While the diabetes online community has a variety of adorably funny memes and videos on the habit of binge-eating during hypoglycemia, it's something we should all take far more seriously.

The long-term consequences are easy to underestimate or miss entirely unless you step back and look at the big picture. Unfortunately, we also don't talk about it at doctor appointments — there's too much shame, and many doctors simply don't realize how often it happens.

Most of them have never experienced low blood sugar and the intense urge to binge that comes with it. They have no idea how common this is when you take insulin to manage diabetes.

Instead, we joke about it. The jokes are often funny, but behind the jokes are real people struggling with a very self-destructive habit that feels like a trap.

In fact, overeating during lows can affect your:

- Self-esteem and confidence
- Mental health (fueling anxiety and depression)
- Ability to manage your weight
- A1c and time-in-range goals
- Long-term diabetes health
- Risk of diabetes complications

- Gut health
- Confidence in managing diabetes
- Energy for the remainder of the day
- Overall energy
- Social life and relationships
- Ability to focus at work, school, etc.
- Total insulin usage
- Self-destructive thoughts and guilt
- Feelings of shame, guilt, embarrassment
- Overall relationship with food

Overeating during lows can also fuel other self-destructive behaviors, including self-harm and disordered eating, like purging or severe calorie restriction in the days after a binge. Severe lows can also increase your risk of more severe lows in the hours that follow because your liver glucose stores are probably very low after that first severe low. It creates a vicious exhausting and dangerous cycle.

This part of your life is so much bigger than simply "eating too much during a low." It's a self-destructive habit. If you step back and truly look at the bigger picture around every binge, you will see a cycle of abuse — but you're the one doing the abusing, and you're the one being abused.

The cycle of abuse: overeating during lows

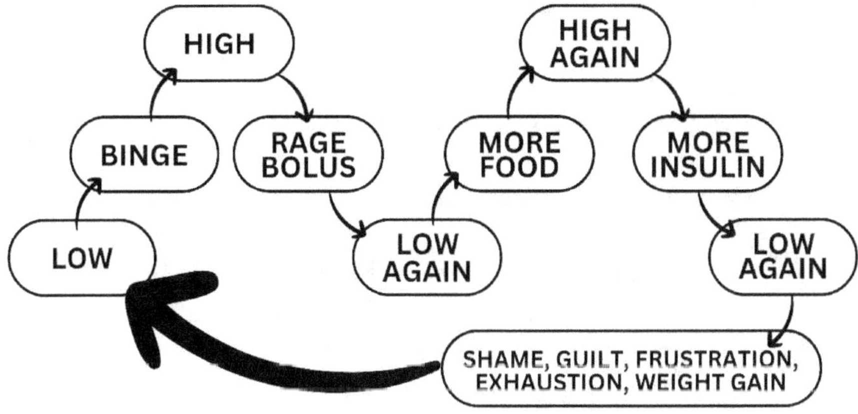

Feels a little dramatic? Let's dig a little deeper.

The calories add up = gradual weight gain

The old school advice is to treat every low blood sugar with 15 grams of carbohydrate. Wait 15 minutes. Check your blood sugar. Treat again with 15 grams if you're still low.

Today, we know some lows only need 5 or 8 grams of carbohydrate. Some lows might need 30 grams. But that's all easier said than done when your brain is begging you to binge.

How many extra calories do you consume every week from overeating during lows?

It adds up. Let's imagine the average binge totals at least 500 calories. Although, we know some hypo binges might add up to 1,000 calories or more. On the conservative side, we'll look at 500 calories per binge.

One binge per week:
- 2,000 extra calories per month
- 24,000 extra calories per year
- Approximately 7 pounds gained per year

Two binges per week:
- 4,000 extra calories per month
- 48,000 extra calories per year
- Approximately 14 pounds gained per year

Three binges per week:
- 6,000 extra calories per month
- 72,000 extra calories per year
- Approximately 20 pounds gained per year

Managing your weight as a person living with diabetes is hard enough. Research has found that 60 percent of people with diabetes are overweight. Insulin is a fat-storage hormone. After using some glucose in your bloodstream for immediate energy, the rest is stored as back-up glucose in your liver and as body fat.

Managing your weight as a person with diabetes is an uphill battle. You're taking injections of a hormone that is inevitably inferior to the stuff your body is supposed to be making for you!

People living with T1D and T2D also produce more liver glucose (glycogen) than non-diabetics because of other hormones your body doesn't produce properly!

This means you need more insulin to manage that excess glucose, which means more glucose is inevitably stored as body fat.

Now, let's add regular binge eating during lows to this weight-management battle. It's brutal.

How many times per week are you binge-eating during lows? How many calories are you consuming during those lows? When you add it up and look at the bigger picture, ignoring the damage and destruction to your overall long-term health is impossible.

The post-binge high & rage-bolus damage

Well, it's inevitable. If you just ate 100+ grams of carbs in 20 minutes, you're probably going to end up with a blood sugar over 250 mg/dL. I don't need to remind you of what high blood sugars do to the precious little blood vessels throughout your fingers, toes, eyes, kidneys — okay, everywhere in your body.

We know high blood sugars aren't great. We've heard it a million times from doctors, mainstream media, your parents, and Aunt Jill at Thanksgiving dinner.

But the threat of that high blood sugar means you're now on a new mission: stop that spike at all costs.

How often does overeating during lows lead you to "rage bolus"?

The term "rage bolus" was created by the always-clever diabetes community. It refers to the moment you give yourself an unreasonably large dose of insulin to correct a high blood sugar — or to cover the 100+ grams of carbs you just ate while binge-eating during a low.

Injectable rapid-acting insulin is so darn slow that the urge to overdose comes easily, even though we know taking more doesn't make it work faster. The rage bolus is usually followed by a dramatic low and, of course, the need to eat more calories.

Binge-eating during lows creates an easy excuse to rage bolus.

- You just ate 100+ grams of carbs
- You know your blood sugar is going to spike dramatically
- You feel guilt and shame over binge-eating
- You feel guilt and shame over the eventual spike in your blood sugar
- You feel guilt and shame when you see 250 mg/dL on your glucometer
- You feel guilt and shame when you see double UP arrows on your CGM
- You take a very large dose of rapid-acting insulin
- You hope it's just the right amount
- You feel anxiety over the potential of going low again
- You eventually see double DOWN arrows on your CGM
- You start eating again to cope with the panic of another potential low

The vicious cycle continues.

Like overeating during lows, rage-bolusing is both self-destructive and a desperate attempt to survive. Lows are scary and immediately life-threatening. Highs carry the worry about damaging your eyes and fingers over decades. Highs look like a "bad diabetic" to anyone who peeks over your shoulder at your glucometer or CGM data. Highs lead to high A1c levels, which lead to feeling like a failure at the doctor's office.

Highs are just as lousy as lows. Rage-bolusing is how you're trying to cope. You're also desperately trying to minimize the guilt that comes with bingeing, hoping to prevent the high. The rage-bolus re-fuels the self-destructive cycle of overeating during lows.

The impact on your energy & daily life

Exhausted? Yeah, that makes sense. The rollercoaster of bingeing during lows is like a big KAPOW on your energy in a few ways.

- **The low blood sugar itself:** Surviving low blood sugar means you just survived your body nearly running out of its primary fuel source! Um, yes, that's going to leave you feeling pretty darn tired even when your blood sugar comes back up.
- **The very full belly:** Overeating during lows leaves you feeling about as energized as Thanksgiving dinner. Your belly is packed. Bleh. Feel like moving much? Bleh. Wanna help your kids with their homework? Bleh. Wanna sit at your desk and work? Bleh. A full belly simply leaves you wanting to take a nap.
- **The quickly rising blood sugar:** Like thick maple syrup trudging slowly through your veins, high blood sugar doesn't leave you feeling "high" with energy. It's just another reason you want to curl up in bed and hide under a thick blanket.

Raise your hand if you have time to feel totally exhausted!

Some exhaustion in life we cannot prevent. Work. Parenting. Taxes. Health insurance. In-laws. That neighbor who fusses over the leaves from *your* tree that fall into *her* yard. And the news, oh dear, the news.

Ask yourself, how does binge eating during low blood sugar affect:

- Your work performance
- Your immediate family members
- Your intimate relationships
- Your social activities

Maybe you're hiding the lows and the overeating from your family? Maybe you avoid social outings or cancel at the last minute after a binge? Maybe the impact on your weight has affected your confidence in your relationships? Maybe you're struggling to keep up with your work some days?

If there's a source of stress in your life that you can actually minimize, that's a big opportunity because you have enough stress.

Binge-eating with low blood sugars may not feel preventable right now — but it will be by the time you finish this book. Minimizing sources of exhaustion in your life is a really good reason to change how you manage low blood sugars.

The shame & embarrassment you carry

Even if you're posting funny memes about it on Instagram, it's still embarrassing and wrought with shame at the moment. And that shame follows you for hours when you're dealing with the aftermath of overeating.

If you're overeating during lows multiple times per week, it's safe to say that shame and guilt become a pestering little thing that lives on your shoulder. You feel guilty that it happened, and you dread when it's going to happen again.

It changes your self-esteem. Your self-worth. In a real way.

Our daily decisions shape us. The less we feel in charge of our decisions, the less confident we feel, the less proud we feel, the less successful we feel. If you feel like you cannot control how much you eat during lows, that feeling will affect your confidence and your pride in every bit of your life.

You feel powerless. This means you eventually feel defeated — over and over every time you binge during a low. It's like diabetes just won another game, and of course, you lost. And you're supposed to show up again tomorrow for another game feeling excited to play? Ugh.

Instead of fueling your confidence — like "Hey, I manage this challenging part of diabetes like a pro!" — binge eating during lows drains your confidence.

It just feels lousy. Over and over.

Ginger's example:

This habit is exhausting. In my mid-20s, I was finally sick of it. I was sick of the aftermath that comes with eating two bowls of cereal, a couple of granola bars, and half a pint of ice cream. I was sick of the shame, the guilt, and the frustration that comes with a blood sugar of 350 mg/dL.

The exhaustion transitions from "dangerously low" to "severely high." I went from feeling panic-stricken, weak, and intensely desperate to feeling completely lethargic.

The super high blood-like-maple-syrup feeling made my brain feel like it was suddenly very depressed or totally shutting down.

I was tired of it. I wanted to change it. Changing it started with simply being honest about it: I am overeating during lows. Big time. I don't need to do this. It doesn't serve me. It's making diabetes harder, not easier. It's not helping me.

It actually feels like I'm hurting myself with food. The damage from that binge takes hours and hours to recover from. It's brutal. I don't want to keep doing this to myself. I'm responsible for how much I eat during any low blood sugar. I can stop myself.

That's where I started.

The truth can be hard to swallow

I realize I haven't exactly painted the most inspiring picture here. Instead, I've painted the truth. Binge-eating during lows is about so much more than just eating too many calories.

The vicious cycle of this habit is real. It is affecting many parts of your life. Next, we'll look at the thoughts in your head that have you convinced there's nothing you can do about it.

Chapter 2

SPOTTING SELF-DESTRUCTIVE HABITS & EXCUSES

Warning: This chapter combines a kick-in-the-butt lecture with cheesy, empowering chit-chat. You need it! Please keep reading. I promise most of the empowering and cheesy chit-chat is contained in this chapter. Mostly.

You've probably been telling yourself for a very long time that you don't have a choice: you have to eat everything during lows. You can't help it. You can't stop it. Your brain is begging you to eat more, and you have to listen.

- You can't stop eating.
- You need to keep eating because your brain wants you to.
- It's a normal part of living with diabetes.
- It's a normal part of taking insulin.
- It's the only option.

Here's a different idea: You DO have control over how much you eat during a low blood sugar.

You're the one putting the food in your mouth. You know you're overeating while you're doing it. You know you'll need insulin to compensate for all those extra carbs. You know you're going to rage-bolus because you feel guilty for over-treating that low before you're even done eating. You know you're setting yourself up for an exhausting day of roller coaster blood sugars.

This is the chapter where we're gonna stop pretending to be helpless.

You are in charge of how much food you eat during any low blood sugar.

If you believe you're helpless, you will be

Every time you tell yourself, "I can't help it, I've gotta keep eating," you are deciding to let your diabetes run your life. It's so much more than too many calories and too many carbohydrates. You're letting diabetes lead to annoying weight gain. You're letting it lead to rage bolusing and a blood sugar roller coaster. You're letting it probably ruin tomorrow, let alone today.

You're letting your diabetes run the show. This is your show!

A big part of taking more ownership over how you treat low blood sugars also gives you more ownership over how you let diabetes affect your life every day.

You are in charge of how much food you eat during a low blood sugar.

Stop giving diabetes power it doesn't actually have. You are the one putting the food in your mouth. You can stop. Your diabetes isn't that powerful. You are in charge. You are not helpless.

Self-pity in diabetes is a trap

Self-pity can be the gasoline, the match, and the fire. Self-pity in diabetes is common — it can fuel overeating during low blood sugars, anger at the A1c that won't budge, or make the daily burden of diabetes feel even heavier.

If you're stuck feeling sorry for yourself because you live with diabetes, you'll be stuck overeating during lows. You'll be stuck with the A1c that's higher than your goal. You'll be stuck feeling like diabetes is always, always, always weighing you down.

This is self-pity. This is your brain overflowing with thoughts and beliefs that life shouldn't be this hard for you. It's unfair. It's not right. It's harder for you than other people.

This is where you'll stay. This is where you'll be stuck. Unless you're up for a new challenge, stop feeling sorry for yourself.

Life is hard — for everyone

Life is hard. It's hard for you. It's hard for your neighbor. It's hard for your brother, your best friend, your boss, and your worst enemy. Nobody gets it easy on this planet. Even Michael Jordan and Taylor Swift face their share of pain, heartbreak, depression, loss, anxiety, stress, and turmoil.

Life is hard.

Diabetes is just one of your challenges. It might be one of the first big challenges in your life, but it won't be the last.

If you live your life often telling yourself that life is unfair for you because of your challenges, this is the same mindset that tells you binge-eating during low blood sugars is completely out of your control.

If you want to ditch the binge-eating, you've gotta start by ditching the self-pity.

Fortunately, it's just a habit. It's really no different than your habit of biting your nails when you're anxious, flossing your teeth before bed, or leaving your dirty socks on the floor next to the laundry bin. It's just a habit.

You can change a habit.

Catch the thoughts that say, "poor me"

How do you change a self-pity habit?

First, be honest about what's in your head. Write it down. What do you keep telling yourself? Write it down.

Next, come up with the message you'd like to put in its place. Something like:

- Life is challenging. I'm here for the challenge.
- Life isn't supposed to be easy! Let's see what I can handle.
- I am going to live a joyful life no matter what.

- This is my life! I will make it what I want it to be.
- I am grateful to be alive! Let's go!
- Another day, another opportunity to make this day count.
- Another challenge? Let's see what I've got.
- Another challenge? I'm gonna give it my best.
- This challenge is not going to stop me.
- I can do this.
- One day at a time.

It may feel cheesy, but you've allowed some pretty icky self-pity thoughts to linger in your head now for years and years. Replacing those icky thoughts with some cheesy positivity seems like a worthwhile trade.

Write that cheesy positivity down in seven different places. Put it on your phone as a daily reminder. Write it on a piece of paper taped to your bathroom mirror. Put it on a note card on the dashboard of your car. Tape it to the coffee machine and your desk at work. Write it on your hand with a permanent marker.

Then, swap out the icky thought when you feel it sneaking in for the cheesy positivity. You have to do the work. You have to reach for the positivity when you feel the icky thought creeping in. You have to stop yourself. You have to resist that cozy feeling of miserable self-pity and reach for the new and uncomfortable positivity instead.

It's a scary thing: ditching the self-pity.

You see, self-pity is the easy way out. Self-pity means you get to blame the universe for what's hard in life. The cheesy positivity means you are owning your life, owning your decisions, and owning your own joy. That can be pretty scary, even if it does sound more fun than miserable self-pity.

You have to keep making that swap for cheesy positivity over miserable self-pity over and over and over. Until one day, the positivity starts popping in naturally. You don't have to reach for it, because it arrived first. That's a new habit.

You are not a victim of diabetes

If you want to change the habit of overeating during lows, you have to ditch the belief that diabetes happened to you and your life now sucks because of it.

You have to choose resilience.

Life is hard for everyone. If you hadn't been served a challenging dish of diabetes, you would've been served a different challenging dish. Nobody gets out of this place easily. If you think someone in your life does have it easy, you simply don't know them very well.

You are not a victim of diabetes. You are a person. You live with diabetes. Diabetes is challenging. Life is challenging. You are here, and you're gonna do your very best to live a full life with diabetes and whatever other challenges life serves up for you — because there will be more.

Your resilience — your ability to endure challenging moments and get back up — is what truly determines your ability to thrive with diabetes. It's not your A1c or your time-in-range, or how many vegetables you eat. It's your resilience. You are resilient!

You are in charge of what you eat

It truly starts with your own thoughts. Here are a few things to reach for during your next low (and to write and tape to your bathroom mirror):

- I am in charge of how much food I eat during this low blood sugar.
- Abusing myself with food during this low blood sugar will not feel good later.
- Abusing myself with food during this low blood sugar will continue to harm me in other ways.
- Abusing myself with food during this low blood sugar is negatively affecting many parts of my life.
- I am in charge of how much insulin I take if I do overeat during this low blood sugar.

- I do not need 50 grams of carbohydrates to treat this low blood sugar.
- I do not need 100 grams of carbohydrates to treat this low blood sugar.
- I do not need 200 grams of carbohydrates to treat this low blood sugar.
- I do not need 300 grams of carbohydrates to treat this low blood sugar.
- I can eat this yummy food when my blood sugar is stable.
- I should try eating 15 grams of fast-acting carbohydrates and wait.
- I'm feeling very, very anxious about this low blood sugar. I'm going to eat 30 grams of carbohydrates thoughtfully, then call a friend and chat with them until I feel safe.
- I am not a victim of diabetes. I am resilient and in charge of my life.
- Life is challenging for everyone. I will face these challenges.
- I am in charge of how much food I eat during this low blood sugar.

These thoughts can become habits even when your blood sugar is 50 mg/dL. You have to choose them, though. You have to ditch the self-pity and choose the cheesy positivity.

Ginger's example:

In addition to everything you just read, I also surrounded myself with positive reinforcements in my early 20s. I'm particularly fond of Bruce Lee and Aristotle, so I wrote empowering quotes from these two gentlemen on notecards and taped them throughout my apartment.

These quotes directly changed how I manage my health and my diabetes:

"You are what you repeatedly do. Excellence, then, is not an act but a habit." - Aristotle

Wanna be the fit, healthy person who exercises every day? Get up and do it. When you're coming up with excuses like "Ugh, I'm tired," get up and do it! You are the person who exercises every day if you make that choice in the moment. Get up and do it. You are the result of the decisions you make over and over.

I don't waste my free time. I make time for the gym, for a jog outside, or a jump rope in the garage. I don't let myself create excuses based on tricky circumstances. I adapt. I figure it out.

"There are no limits. There are only plateaus, and you must not stay there, you must go beyond them." - Bruce Lee

I learned to see myself as a constant work in progress without any limits! My relationship with food even ten years ago is so different than my relationship with food today because I gave myself the space to keep evolving and learning. My knowledge of my own diabetes is significantly greater today because I never stopped asking questions and trying to learn more. The moment you think you've learned it all is when you stop evolving, stop improving, and stop growing.

"What you habitually think largely determines what you ultimately become." - Bruce Lee

I am responsible for putting good thoughts in my head. What I allow myself to think every day leads to everything else! If you're telling yourself you're not good enough, you will continue to let yourself down, fail to meet your goals, and feel like you're not good enough.

Take responsibility for your own thoughts. Put good thoughts in there! "I am good enough. I am capable of managing my relationship with food! I can reach my A1c goals if I keep learning and keep trying."

"Knowing is not enough; we must apply. Willing is not enough; we must do." - Bruce Lee

You're low, and you know you only need 10 grams of carbs. This is the moment when you get to dig deep and apply what you know instead of giving in to your urge to eat everything.

It's those little moments that count. The little decisions. The decision to get up and walk at 6 a.m. or keep sleeping. The decision to order the easy takeout pizza or go home and prepare your own dinner with real, fresh ingredients. The decision to eat one slice of cake at the party or three slices of cake.

It's not about being perfect. It's about holding yourself accountable for those little decisions.

Resilience is your strength

Resilience is a fancy word for the idea that you are surviving no matter what challenges life keeps throwing at you.

Although we've never met, I have a pretty good hunch that you aren't giving yourself enough credit for your resilience and strength. Every single day, diabetes is trying to hold you back. Every single day, diabetes is trying to kill you. Yup, I said it. (I'm kind of blunt sometimes.) Whether you have type 1 or type 2, diabetes is trying to kill you quickly, slowly, or both.

And here you are! You showed up for another day! If I could include swears in this book, I'd definitely include one right here! $%&#! You are here for another day! Give yourself some credit for this accomplishment.

This is how people who are overflowing with confidence and self-esteem pull it off. They talk themselves up. They acknowledge their strengths. They acknowledge their hard work even if the results weren't perfect — even if they failed.

So, your blood sugar was high all day? Well, that means you endured high blood sugars all day long while dealing with every other responsibility in your life!

So, you forgot to take insulin at lunch? Who wouldn't forget this on occasion? You're supposed to take insulin every single time you eat? Have you ever explained that to a non-diabetic and watched their jaw drop? That's not an easy thing to ask of anyone.

So, you ate an entire pizza when you were really stressed out last night? Okay. Guess what? That was one moment. You are made up of a million moments.

This moment (the one with the pizza) doesn't define you. It's just how you choose to manage your stress that day. You might do it again next week. You're human. You might choose differently next time if you want to. But you are more than that moment.

So, you've been skipping some of your insulin doses? Well, who could blame you? It isn't fun taking this medication every single day.

But it sounds like you're struggling, and you could use some extra support. It sounds like you might need to remind yourself that you deserve extra support and that it's okay to ask for help. It sounds like life feels extra hard for you right now, and this is how you're trying to cope, control, or just simply survive. You're dealing with a lot.

You are very resilient. The fact that you're still alive to read this book tells me that you are one heck of a human being. Like most humans, you've got some flaws and weaknesses. You've got some fears. You've got some habits that aren't helping you.

But that doesn't change the fact that you are very, very resilient. And you probably deserve more credit than you're giving yourself for how much you endure every single day.

Chapter 3

LET'S TALK ABOUT PANIC & STRESS

To change how you manage your eating habits during low blood sugars, we've gotta talk about the panic that often comes with those lows.

I think we can all agree that most people don't usually make great decisions while panicking. Instead, panic is when we tend to lose control and do things we wouldn't normally do — like eat a whole carton of ice cream and three bowls of cereal in 30 minutes.

There are a whole bunch of really good reasons to panic during hypoglycemia. In fact, your CGM pretty much tells you to panic when it's alarming, flashing red, and showing double-down arrows. We all know those arrows aren't pointing down towards good things.

To save your own life, diabetes wants you to panic. And that's really what's happening when you binge. You are panicking. I don't blame you. But if you panic every time you're low or even half the time when you're low, you're gonna find yourself overeating pretty darn often, then struggling with the consequences of overeating all the time.

It's important to realize and say to yourself, "Hey, I am full of panic right now." The moment you identify what you're feeling is the moment you can also say, "Hey, you don't need to panic. You don't need to eat everything in sight. Take a deep breath. You're gonna be okay. Just treat the low."

In this chapter, let's look at the stress and panic in diabetes a little closer. This isn't a fun place to shine a spotlight. I get it. But you can't change it if you don't look at it.

Alarms + Arrows = Anxiety

Low blood sugars can be very scary. Did I mention that already? But these days, it's not just the lows that trigger panic and anxiety. Now we have arrows and alarms — BEEP BEEP BEEP — to warn us of the impending danger! BEEP BEEP BEEP. That sound is telling you: Eat! Survive! Eat! Survive! Eat!

Low blood sugars induce panic for a good reason: your body wants you to take action. But that panic can leak into your entire day. It can almost become a new mode you're operating in all day. To live at that level of worry all day long — calling that "stressful" is an understatement.

Today's technology has completely changed your daily safety and ability to manage tighter blood sugar levels with diabetes. Yes, it warns you of oncoming lows during exercise, while you're driving, when you're sleeping, and every moment in between. We are all safer thanks to this technology.

But those arrows and alarms can also fuel panic and anxiety.

It's a tricky double-edged sword: you can't get the same protection from hypoglycemia if you turn the alarms off, but simply seeing those arrows or hearing that alarm can trigger overeating, too.

Maybe you never even noticed: are the arrows and alarms on your CGM contributing to your overeating during lows?

- The audible alerts interrupt your morning, your workday, your sleep, your child's piano concert, and your workout. Yes, those are much-needed alerts, but they are disruptive. The mere sound tells you to panic and take action. It's a double-edged sword.
- The visual alerts of down arrows fuel anxiety because you don't know just how low that arrow is indicating. The arrow can also turn sideways at the next reading in five minutes, completely changing the degree of concern and alarm.

The more aware you are of how your CGM is fueling anxiety and panic, the more you can manage it, stay ahead of it, and talk yourself through it.

Here are a few questions to ask yourself:

- **Treating lows that were never gonna happen:** Do you start eating when you see a DOWN arrow even when you're not low yet? At what blood sugar level with down arrows do you tend to start eating? Are you treating down arrows at 120 mg/dL that might have never dropped below 80 mg/dL?
- **Treating arrows instead of lows:** Are you eating until you see the arrows turn sideways despite the known 15-minute delay between your blood sugar level and the number on your CGM? Speaking of 15, when's the last time you ate just 15 grams of carbs, waited 15 minutes, then rechecked your blood glucose before eating another 15 grams? (Then you see the UP arrows and rage bolus? Eeesh, the roller coaster begins.)
- **Arrows can turn quickly:** Do you ever see a slanted down arrow with an in-range blood glucose level that suddenly becomes a sideways arrow five minutes later? But you already started treating the arrow, not the number. It feels like a trick, but it's the reality of today's technology. It's not perfect.

If you find yourself doing any of the above, it's time to create new goals for how you react to those arrows. I use the word "goals" because it suggests you're striving towards something rather than suddenly doing it perfectly starting tomorrow. For example:

- "I will not treat arrows. I will treat the numbers."
- "I will eat 15 grams, wait 15 minutes, then check again before treating again."
- "I will only eat more than 15 grams of carbohydrates if the arrows suggest I'm headed towards severe hypoglycemia."

We'll add these little goals to your new guidelines for treating lows in Chapter 5.

There's no doubt that CGM technology is preventing and reducing your risk of severe hypoglycemia. CGMs might also reduce our own physical awareness of oncoming low blood sugars.

You might not notice unless you take a break from your CGM, but there's a good chance your own physical awareness of hypo symptoms has relaxed since you started wearing this tech.

And it makes sense — you know your CGM will beep at you if you go low, so that little protection part of your brain has relaxed. This is really an intended part of wearing a CGM, right? To help you relax a little? But, the long-term result is that you might not be feeling those early and subtle low symptoms as much.

That doesn't mean you should stop using it. It's just something to keep in mind.

Breaking news: diabetes is stressful

Before adding low blood sugars to the mix, diabetes is plenty stressful. You already know this. But you might not know that the medical world has actually legitimized and named the kind of stress you experience every single day. Actually, there are a few new medical terms I want you to know about — because they validate everything you feel.

- Diabetes distress
- Fear of hypoglycemia (FoH)

The fact that these are now official medical terms should tell you a few things.

First, you are not alone. This blood sugar circus you're juggling every day is not easy for anyone. Secondly, simply taking a minute to acknowledge just how much stress you endure every single day can, a little bit, lighten that stress. When you get to truly acknowledge something versus trying to endure silently, it can change the feeling of that stress.

When you find yourself frustrated, exhausted, or anxious in any given moment of diabetes, remember that how you feel is valid, but it's also *normal* because any type of this disease is really stressful, especially if you take insulin.

When you find yourself struggling, remind yourself that the struggle is normal. Give yourself a little more credit for what you endure. Cut yourself a little more slack for struggling sometimes. Instead of beating yourself up, talk yourself up: "This is really hard, and I'm waking up every day to deal with it again. I am a very resilient human being!"

Diabetes distress

- Defined as "the unique, often hidden emotional burdens and worries that are part of the spectrum of patient experience when managing a severe, demanding chronic disease like diabetes," according to research from the University of California, San Francisco, published in *Diabetes Care*.

Diabetes distress is a cute name for the non-stop work of managing a disease that requires hour-by-hour attention, can be life-threatening at any moment, and involves daily medication management. Medications that are tedious, inexact, dangerous, and expensive. Okay, I'll stop there.

You've got carb-counting, medications, insulin injections, blood sugar levels, finger pricks, CGM sensors, insulin pump infusion sites, more carb-counting, the guilt from highs, the fear of lows, the doctor appointments, the eye exams, and the worry or reality of diabetes complications.

Don't forget the lectures from family, friends, strangers, and mainstream media. The dismissive (and usually inaccurate) comments in movies and comedy. The judgy comments from your healthcare team (unless you fired them already and found a better team).

The hours and hours you waste every year trying to convince your health insurance company that you still need insulin, test strips, CGMs, and insulin pump supplies. The thousands of dollars you spend on life-saving supplies.

Yes, you can justifiably claim to feel a bit of stress. A bit of diabetes distress.

If your diabetes distress, however, is affecting your ability to get through your day, then it's probably time to ask for help.

Please consider talking to your healthcare team immediately If diabetes distress is:
- Fueling overall depression and/or anxiety
- Preventing you from managing the daily tasks of diabetes to keep yourself out of the hospital
- Preventing you from managing the daily tasks of diabetes that affect your immediate or long-term safety
- Preventing you from socializing with friends and family
- Preventing you from participating in normal hobbies and activities
- Driving harmful behaviors in your relationship with food
- Contemplating any type of self-harm

All the research says people living with diabetes are significantly more likely to experience depression and anxiety — you are not alone. But, you've gotta speak up and ask for help to get help.

Fear of hypoglycemia (FoH)
- Defined as "a specific and extreme fear evoked by the risk and/or occurrence of low blood glucose levels" by the American Diabetes Association's Mental Health workbook.

You might know FoH as simply running your blood sugars higher in order to reduce your chance of going low. You might know FoH as treating blood sugar levels between 70 to 130 mg/dL with carbohydrates because you're terrified of dropping any lower.

You might know FoH as having woken up after a severe hypoglycemic event — one that led to a seizure or loss of consciousness — and now you're desperate to make sure that never happens again.

Low blood sugars are really scary. Most people who take insulin could probably be diagnosed with FoH, but there is a certain point when it becomes an issue that calls for a bit more attention.

Various research on FoH says it can lead to the following:
- Consistently higher blood sugar levels
- Consistently higher A1c levels
- Higher levels of daily anxiety, depression, diabetes distress
- Higher risk of experiencing diabetic ketoacidosis (DKA)
- Higher risk of developing diabetes-related complications
- More difficulty managing your weight
- Generally decreased quality of life

While FoH is a common part of life if you take insulin, it shouldn't be threatening your immediate and long-term health. That's when it's worth getting more support.

A big part of addressing FoH is working with a diabetes educator and/or therapist to help you:

- Gradually rebuild your confidence in managing low blood sugars — especially after experiencing severe hypoglycemia. This is a bit-by-bit process of relearning that you are capable of managing most low blood sugars safely and effectively.
- Learn deeper insulin management skills to help prevent you from taking too much and improve the accuracy of your doses. Your body's insulin needs can fluctuate throughout your entire life. If you don't adjust your insulin doses, you'll find yourself experiencing scary lows and frustrating highs. (More on that in this book, too!)
- Addressing "hypoglycemia unawareness," which can develop in people who've experienced frequently severe low blood sugar events or in people who've simply lived with diabetes for a very long time. Hypoglycemia unawareness means you no longer feel the noticeable warning signs of low blood sugar. Working with your healthcare team to compensate for this can include getting on a CGM if you aren't already, getting a Diabetes Alert Dog, and other approaches.

It starts by asking for help! Don't deal with FoH on your own.

Ginger's example:

Talk yourself up, baby! This is what I learned to do, and it helps me manage low blood sugars. I talk myself through the panic. That skill applies to panic or anxiety outside of diabetes, too.

When I'm low, yes, I remind myself, "You are in charge of how much you eat during this low. You can handle this low. You are going to be okay. Take a deep breath. You are going to be okay."

When I'm stressed with too much work on my plate, I remind myself, "You're just one gal! You can only do as much as you can do, and that's okay. You've always gotten it done in the past, right? You'll get it done this time. Take a deep breath and just do what you can do."

I talk myself through it. Over and over. And then again. As much as I need to.

The worry & the panic is real

If you take insulin, worrying will be a part of your daily life. You don't vacuum the house, go to the grocery store, or walk your dog without worrying and preparing for low blood sugars.

Talking yourself through the worry and the panic on a daily basis is part of what makes you so resilient, and it's a skill you need to keep developing until they find a cure.

Chapter 4

Your relationship with food plays a big role in how you manage food during low blood sugars. When you're constantly trying to follow strict diets, low blood sugars become the perfect opportunity to finally eat the food you've been restricting.

For most people, those super strict diets are a yo-yo part of their life — you follow it for a few days or weeks, rebound, then try to get back on that super strict diet. Round and round. The opportunity to binge when you're low contributes to that round-and-round yo-yo cycle.

Instead, if you create a "diet" that includes space for those foods — where no food is "bad," "evil," or off-limits — then you don't need to abuse them during low blood sugars. You can just let yourself eat those foods and actually enjoy eating them when your blood sugar is sitting pretty at 120 mg/dL.

Easier said than done. Let's get started.

Twisted up from the moment you're diagnosed

Type 1 and type 2 diabetes affects your entire relationship with food from the moment you're diagnosed. It changes everything. And that relationship affects how you treat lows, too — but we'll get to that in a bit.

In many ways, the impact on your relationship with food can be positive. You've learned intense details about nutrition that most people around you never will. You might've learned tremendous discipline around food because of diabetes. You are more in tune with how any snack, meal, or beverage affects your body because of diabetes.

But that hyper-focus on food can twist your relationship with food, too.

You have to count every gram of carbohydrate. Every crumb. And along the way, you inevitably learn the calories, fat, and protein in everything you eat. No meal can ever be relaxing or carefree. Every meal is work because you have to calculate insulin doses.

From the moment you're diagnosed, your doctor, your family, and society start lecturing you about everything you eat! These foods are "bad," and those foods are "good," and you're "bad" if you eat these foods, and you're "good" if you eat those foods.

It's exhausting.

When T1D twists your relationship with food

Over time, how you cope with that hyper-focus on food can turn into some not-so-great habits and a very self-destructive relationship with food.

It might look like:

- Binge-eating during low blood sugars because you can finally eat some of the foods you usually try to avoid and restrict
- Avoiding certain foods for days or weeks to the point of deprivation, then binge-eating those foods for days
- Avoiding entire food groups (like all carbs) for days or weeks, then binge-eating that food group for days
- Constantly stopping and starting restrictive diets that leave you feeling deprived and eventually binge-eating
- Developing an eating disorder, like anorexia or bulimia
- Skipping insulin (diabulimia) which can be life-threatening
- Purposefully overdosing insulin so you have an excuse to binge

But listen, this doesn't have to be how it goes forever. It is possible to change your relationship with food completely. It is possible to break free from this exhausting, self-destructive relationship with food and find some peace! It is possible to create a relationship with food that leaves you feeling like you are in charge, satisfied, and empowered by your decisions around food.

Let's dig a little deeper.

Pressure. Pressure. Pressure.

It's everywhere. The pressure to "eat this, not that" is present even for people who produce plenty of insulin, but those of us with any type of diabetes feel it extra. Like whoa.

It's in the news. It's in stand-up comedy. It's in movies (but usually portrayed totally wrong). It's at the doctor's office. Your mom's house. Your aunt's Thanksgiving. Your grandpa's worried eyebrows when you grab a cookie at Sunday dinner. It's at school. It's with friends at restaurants who haven't learned enough about diabetes yet. It's with well-meaning in-laws. It's on social media. It's everywhere.

A lot of what we're told contradicts other stuff we're told.

Friends, doctors, and family hate it when your diet is too strict, but they love to freak out when you eat pizza and a cupcake.

Your doctor doesn't want you on a controversial ketogenic diet, but you can also feel judged for eating practically anything else! Even the pamphlets you can find are confusing and contradicting: eat more brown rice — oh, but limit starch. Don't eat dessert, but don't try to be perfect. Huh? What? Ugh.

- Cut the carbs. (But get enough grains?)
- Eat less meat.
- Eat more protein. (Oh, but less meat?)
- Dietary fat is good for you! (Oh, wait, but not that fat!)
- Eat mostly carbs. (Except not too many carbs.)
- Only eat plants. (But you need milk and meat, too!)
- Drink this diet product thing. (But then eat more real food!)
- Eat this fake sugar product thing. (But wait, eat more real food!)
- Take this medicine — it will help! (Hey, that's cheating!)

- Always eat breakfast.
- Try skipping breakfast…and lunch!
- Never eat dessert. Dessert is bad.
- Eat dessert sometimes…you need balance!
- Don't follow a diet. (But try following this diet.)

All you're left with is steamed broccoli and real chicken.

It's time to tune out the noise. Like Bruce Lee said, "Take what is useful and leave the rest."

Create your personal guidelines around food

This next part takes some work. Some self-experimenting. Some letting go of old icky diet habits that have never actually helped you, but you keep doing them over and over.

The "perfect diet" is not out there in the universe for you. The "perfect diet" is something you need to create for yourself.

A few things to consider:
- **More whole foods:** How much of your breakfast, lunch, or dinner contains whole fruit, nuts, beans, non-processed meat, and vegetables? It doesn't have to be 100%. A big salad with veggies, chicken, and salad dressing is still mostly whole food!
- **Fewer processed foods:** How many times a day do you reach for processed, packaged stuff? Your "perfect diet" doesn't have to include zero of these items, but maybe it's something you limit to once or twice per day.
- **Yummy things you love:** When you declare all chocolate or all bread as "evil" and try to avoid it, don't you just end up obsessed with it? Instead, maybe it's time to plan for it in your day! Make space for it. Allow yourself to eat a thoughtful serving of it every day or every few days to prevent deprivation. Then, it won't control you. It has less power.
- **Buy the food you often binge eat:** What if you just bought 7 of the food you usually binge on? 7 candy bars or 7 pints of ice cream? What if there was so much of it in your freezer that you couldn't possibly binge and eat it all in one night?

- **Suddenly, it's not so powerful.** It's just there in your freezer. Maybe you could enjoy a thoughtful serving without the pressure of trying to get rid of it. Without the pressure of trying to eat it all because it's going to be off-limits for the next nine weeks?
- **Be realistic, too.** To lose weight or manage your weight, limiting calories to a certain extent is usually necessary. Most people cannot simply eat whatever they want without weight gain, blood sugar woes, and an impact on their health. Your daily diet needs to include some restraint and limits to serve your goals. That doesn't mean it needs to be perfect!

Food is so personal, but so is eating. Some people feel great after eating a big breakfast! Some people feel totally bogged down by breakfast and appreciate fasting until I p.m.! Which one are you?

As you create your own "perfect diet," ask yourself a few questions:

- **What parts of that trendy low-carb diet worked well for you?** There's plenty to learn from any fad diet. For example, while trying to cut carbs, maybe you discovered a few low-carb meals you enjoy. Maybe you found eating low-carb at breakfast easier, but you craved carbs at night? Use that information to shape when you eat carbs.
- **What did you learn about how your body responds to certain foods?** Does oatmeal for breakfast make you feel energized or groggy? Does a big meal at lunch trigger cravings for dessert all afternoon? Does that tiny salad leave you feeling desperately hungry by dinner and you end up binge-eating at 8 p.m.? Do you feel good after eating fast food?
- **What foods bring you joy?** Include it carefully — even if it's French fries or chocolate or pasta. Food is meant to be joyful! Just because you have diabetes doesn't mean you can't enjoy those more indulgent foods. But there's gotta be thought and balance to it. That means making space for it in your day. Planning for it. The more you eat it with intention, the less it will control you, the less you will feel the urge to binge, and the more you will enjoy eating it.

This is your own diet science project! Try new things. Let yourself experiment — and potentially fail. You might overeat ice cream one day. That's okay. Think about what led to the ice cream binge. Ask yourself how it felt. And next time, try eating a more moderate amount.

You know the restrictive yo-yo dieting thing doesn't work for you. Try something different: remove all the rules and create your own guidelines.

Guidelines aren't rules

Guidelines aren't rules. They're more like the bumpers in a bowling alley. They're meant to help you be aware of your goals without everything being so black and white or "perfect vs. fail." While you're creating your own guidelines around food, stay self-aware.

Ask yourself: how do I feel? What old beliefs and habits keep trying to pry their way in? What do I really want my relationship with food to look like?

Ginger's example:

Here are examples of my personal guidelines for nutrition that help me reach my diabetes and health goals without too much restriction. These guidelines leave me feeling empowered and in charge of my decisions around food. These guidelines allow me to enjoy the stereotypically "healthy" foods and the not-so-perfect foods.

- I feel best when following a 16:8 intermittent fasting schedule, which means I skip breakfast and eat my first meal around noon or 1 p.m.
- I feel best when my first meal is a big salad with veggies, full-fat salad dressing, some nuts, and some whole fruit.
- I feel best when I drink only one cup of coffee in the morning, then water and seltzer the rest of the day.
- I feel best when I stop working at 3 p.m. and remember to eat a light snack like gluten-free toast with butter and sea salt or raw veggies with hummus or an apple with peanut butter.

- I feel best when I eat mostly lighter, cold foods during the day.
- I get really bogged down by hot, big meals for lunch. No bueno.
- I feel best when I avoid sugary or heavy foods during the day.
- I feel best when I eat vegetarian during the day.
- I feel best when I eat meat and a variety of veggies for dinner.
- I feel best when I save my starchiest carb choices for an evening dessert.
- I feel best when I limit my alcohol consumption to the weekend.
- I sleep best with a full stomach. I do not sleep well if I'm hungry.
- French fries make me feel sick. They ruin my sleep. They disturb my happiness even into the next day! Dear self: try not to eat French fries very often. (Please, and thank you.)

This is what I know about my body, energy, cravings, and what I need to maintain a positive relationship with food. These are all conclusions I've come to through experimenting with judgment. Then, take what is useful and leave the rest.

You might notice, too, that none of these guidelines are rules. None of these guidelines say, "I cannot eat ______ ever," or "I cannot eat ____ during the day."

If I want to veer from these guidelines, that's my choice! It's up to me! It doesn't mean I've failed, it just means I didn't follow my own guidelines that day.

Sometimes, on the weekends, I purposefully break from these guidelines, and I eat gluten-free pancakes for breakfast covered in syrup. By the time Monday arrives, I'm desperate for my guidelines because I never feel great after eating pancakes, even if they are delicious.

Most of the time, I choose to follow these guidelines because I know I feel best when I do. When I don't follow them, I don't feel as good and my blood sugars are harder to manage.

Change it up with simple experiments

Think of your personal guidelines as a big giant experiment. It doesn't have to be this tremendously perfect plan on day one. It can start small with one part of the day or one type of food. Keep it simple.

For example, you could start with *one* of these ideas:

- Try eating vegetables and protein/fat for breakfast instead of processed carbs.
- Try giving yourself permission to eat ice cream every single night this week instead of trying so hard to avoid it.
- Try limiting your caffeine consumption to a certain amount, then switching to water.
- Try eating more raw vegetables at lunch instead of bread.
- Try grabbing fruit and nuts instead of the bag of chips at 3 p.m.
- Try drinking a big glass of water as soon as you wake up.
- Try learning how to saute broccoli and onions for dinner.
- Try eliminating diet soda for one week and drinking water or seltzer instead.
- Try giving yourself permission to eat bread at dinner.
- Try challenging all the rules that have twisted your relationship with food.

This process doesn't happen overnight. You don't need to have a solid list of guidelines in place by next month! It can take months and years. The most important part is to be honest with yourself and try new things.

I knew a gal once who said, "Well, I'm all or nothing," to justify why she kept stopping and starting extremely restrictive diets. She was certain that was the only approach that could work for her. She couldn't see that she was constantly stopping and starting — while eating a lot loaves of bread in between. This reveals that it wasn't actually working for her at all. She couldn't sustain it.

Get out of your own way. Be honest with yourself. And try things you haven't tried before.

Ginger's example:

I was in high school when my "secret eating" behavior started. It was fueled by two things: First, an intrinsic desire to rebel just a little bit against the "rules" of diabetes nutrition. Second, it was the start of a not-so-healthy coping mechanism for stress.

I worked at a movie theater as a projectionist and assistant manager — I was often the last person to leave the theater just before midnight. By the time I got home, the rest of my family was sound asleep.

Some nights, I'd use this time to eat something I "shouldn't" — like dessert. No one in my family was telling me I couldn't eat dessert, but the pressure of diabetes itself left me feeling like it was off-limits. Instead of going to bed, I'd consume another 400+ calories that I probably didn't need. I was already a bit overweight, and this new late-night habit certainly didn't help.

The consequences were just weight gain and shame. It also drained my confidence — but I could only see that clearly years later when I'd overcome this habit and felt so much pride in being in charge of my relationship with food. This little overeating habit quietly picked away my self-esteem, pride, confidence, and feeling of being in charge of my own life.

By college — when stress is bigger and more "real world" compared to high school — my late-night eating and bingeing increased dramatically. Now, I had total privacy in my apartment. In one short drive, I could grab Chinese takeout, a pint of ice cream, and a box of those delicious chocolate iced gluten-loaded doughnuts found in most gas stations.

All the forbidden foods that I knew required loads of insulin and would inevitably leave my blood sugar in the high 200's or 300s. (This was before CGMs existed, by the way. It was easier to ignore the data!) It was my not-so-helpful escape from the stress and anxiety I wasn't facing and didn't know how to deal with.

I gained weight. I felt miserable. My A1c spiked a full point from

7 to 8 percent. I did not feel in charge of my own life.

The first thing I did to change this habit? I owned it. I wrote it down. I described it. I looked at it. I repeatedly told myself, "This isn't helping you." Over and over and over. There is no way out but through. This is tiring. Then, I started thinking about food differently.

Instead of, "I shouldn't eat that or that or that,"...I changed it to, "Actually, I can eat whatever I want. I'm the one who puts that food in my mouth. I can choose anything. Nothing is off limits. There are no rules. There are just my choices."

That doesn't mean I chose all vegetables for the rest of my life. It means I took responsibility for every choice I made.

- "If I choose the box of doughnuts, I'm going to feel like garbage."
- "If I choose to make myself some veggies and chicken, I'm gonna feel pretty good."
- "I am going to enjoy a slice of gluten-free chocolate cake. That's my choice."

Being honest with myself. Taking responsibility for my choices. Being in charge of my relationship with food.

Be your own diet boss

Don't let food boss you around. Being in charge of your relationship with food doesn't mean being "in control" or being perfect. It simply means being the one making the decisions and owning your decisions. If you're gonna eat a pint of ice cream for dinner, fine. Just be honest with yourself about it.

"I'm gonna eat this pint of ice cream for dinner. I'm not gonna feel great after, but I'm not gonna beat myself up for it. And tomorrow is a new day."

Then move on. Tomorrow, you probably won't want to eat a pint of ice cream for dinner.

Chapter 5

TREATING LOWS WITH NEW GUIDELINES

Here's the part where you design your own set of guidelines to help you treat lows thoughtfully and carefully.

You can lean on these guidelines every single time you're low by asking yourself, "Okay, should I go to the kitchen and eat three bowls of cereal and a chocolate bar? Or...should I sit down with the 15 grams of fast-acting carbs I use for lows, then chug a glass of cold water?"

Just like the huge variety of little messages in your head that shape how you treat people, how you perform your tasks at work, how you turn your homework in on time, how you put the dirty dishes in the dishwasher, and pick up after your dog, these guidelines should be tucked in an easy-to-grab spot in your brain.

You'll reach for these guidelines every time you're low.

Let's take a look at a few guidelines to help stop the binge, then you'll create your own.

Stop the binge during hypoglycemia

You know your habits and your weaknesses best, right? You probably know that opening the refrigerator or the cereal cupboard during a 2 a.m. low is not a great idea.

All the yogurt and a whole lotta cereal down the hatch in a matter of minutes. Roller coaster, rage bolusing, guilt, frustration, and exhaustion will follow.

Instead, here are a few guidelines that can prevent the opportunity for binge eating.

It *starts* with the simple "rule of 15"

Just in case you never learned this when you were first prescribed insulin, you should know about the "rule of 15."

- **What "diabetes management 101" says:** Eat 15 grams of fasting-acting carbohydrates. Wait 15 minutes. Recheck your blood sugar. Eat another 15 grams of carbohydrates if needed.
- **What real life with diabetes says:** Most lows need about 15 grams of carbohydrates. Some only need 8. Some need 30 grams. Occasionally, there's a low that needs 60 grams if your insulin dose gets all funky for any given reason.

Even though it's important, it's also obnoxiously simplified as though choosing just 15 grams of carbohydrates is an easy thing to do when you're shaking and sweating during a low.

Regardless, it's a good reminder that most lows require very few carbohydrates — and bingeing will lead to rebound highs.

Don't use yummy food you love to treat lows

Low blood sugar shouldn't be your chance to finally enjoy that ice cream bar. Like we talked about earlier in the book, give yourself space to enjoy that food when your blood sugar is stable, and you can dose insulin for it thoughtfully.

Also, those high-fat foods take significantly longer to break down and digest, which means they take longer to raise your blood sugar! Piling 20 grams of fat into your belly with any carbohydrate is going to dramatically slow down how long it takes for your blood sugar to come back up.

Instead, trying choosing fast-acting carbohydrates you don't mind but don't love — foods you don't *want* to eat tons of. Specifically, fast-acting carbohydrates that break down quickly and raise your blood sugar quickly.

Did you know glucose tabs are the fastest at raising your blood sugar because they're made with dextrose? Dextrose is the only type of sugar that is chemically identical to the glucose in your bloodstream. That means your body doesn't have to spend any time converting dextrose into glucose. Other types of sugar, like sucrose (table sugar) or corn syrup, take longer to break down — which means they take longer to raise your blood sugar. Which means you'll feel lousy for longer, too.

Examples of fast-acting carbohydrates sweetened with dextrose (with zero fat or protein) include:

- Glucose tabs or gel
- BottleCaps
- Smarties (the USA version)
- SweetTarts
- Nerds
- PixieStix
- FunDip

Next on the list are examples of fast-acting carbohydrates that contain other types of sugar, but they're still pretty speedy:.

- Jelly beans
- Fruit snack gummies
- Gummy bears
- Gummy LifeSavers
- Skittles
- Starburst
- Swedish Fish
- Sour Patch Kids
- Candy corn
- Juice or soda
- Marshmallows

What about dried fruit and fresh fruit? These wholesome sources of carbohydrates take even longer to break down because of the fiber and nutrients.

It's certainly better than a chocolate bar, cheese crackers, or ice cream, but definitely not better than fast-acting non-fat candy.

Use foods you can measure carefully

Drinking sips from a bottle of juice can be risky. It's easy to consume 30 grams of carbohydrates instead of 15 grams when you're just sipping.

When you choose specific candies, you can carefully measure how many grams of carbohydrate you're consuming. Most lows only need about 8 to 15 grams of carbohydrates — unless you took way too much insulin and you're continuing to crash.

Learning how to carefully count and track how many carbohydrates you eat carefully is totally possible during a low blood sugar when you remind yourself, "I control how much food I eat during this low."

For example, here are approximate carb-counts for various candies:

- 4 Starburst: 16 grams
- 15 Jelly Belly jelly beans: 15 grams
- 4 Candy corn: 16 grams
- 4 Gummy LifeSavers: 16 grams
- 15 Skittles: 15 grams
- 1 Pouch Welch's Fruit Snacks: 16 grams
- 2 Regular Marshmallows: 12 grams
- 3 Sour Patch Kids: 15 grams
- 7 Mini Swedish Fish: 15 grams

When you choose foods you can carefully measure, you can hold yourself accountable for how much you're consuming during any low blood sugar. Plus, these choices don't really freeze or melt in extreme temperatures — so they'll be easy and safe to eat regardless of how long they sit in your desk, car, or jacket pocket.

Also, I challenge you to think of these foods as "low medicine" rather than candy. These are foods you reach for specifically when you're low. This is the medicine for lows just like you'd grab ibuprofen for a headache or a bandaid for a cut.

These become your "medicine" options for treating lows.

Are there low blood sugars that call for a mega dose of carbohydrates? Yes. We've all had those lows — when you seriously overdosed for a meal, or you took the wrong type of insulin, or exercised with way too much insulin on board. We'll talk about those lows and how to treat them in a minute.

Talk yourself through the CGM arrows anxiety

Remember your goals from Chapter 3 regarding the arrows on your CGM. If you've been in a habit of letting arrows fuel panic and anxiety, it's time to reset how you talk yourself through it:

- "I will not treat arrows. I will treat the numbers."
- "I will eat 15 grams, wait 15 minutes, then check again before treating again."
- "I will only eat more than 15 grams of carbohydrates if the arrows suggest I'm headed towards severe hypoglycemia."

The arrows are meant to keep you safe. Don't let them sabotage your success! Treating or preventing the low is step 1. Step 2 is all about preventing those rebounding highs. You've gotta keep both in the forefront of your mind when you see those stressful arrows.

Are you responding to the rising arrows with too much insulin? Are you a roller coaster operator at the country fair? You're the only person who can stop this vicious cycle. You've got to resist the urge to over-correct the high with a rage bolus of insulin. Take a deep breath and be thoughtful. (Remember, a rising arrow can change directions at any moment!)

Distract yourself for 15 minutes

Your brain doesn't really care how responsible you were when you carefully counted those jelly beans. Your brain still wants more. It's begging you for more. It's painting images of food in your brain, plates and bowls of delicious piles of carbohydrates — trying to lure you to the kitchen.

But you are in control of how much you eat this low, remember? This is when you've gotta dig deep and distract that "Feed me!

Feed me!" with something else.

Here are a few distractions that work for me:

- Drink a tall glass of ice-cold water
- Chew a stick (or two) of gum
- Chew on raw baby carrots or celery
- Set a timer for 10 minutes, lie down, and close your eyes
- Sit on your hands and listen to three of your favorite songs
- GET OUT OF THE KITCHEN
- Seriously, get out of the kitchen as quickly as possible

Keep your "low medicine" stashed everywhere

Visiting the kitchen at 2 a.m. during a low blood sugar is a terrible idea. It's much riskier than visiting the kitchen at 2 p.m. For some reason, that quiet darkness in the middle of the night creates the most wonderful environment for binge-eating everything in sight.

Even better, nobody's gonna witness how much you ate! Secret binge!

This is why you've really gotta avoid the kitchen during lows in the middle of the night. Preparing for lows means putting little bags of "low medicine" in all the right places and replenishing those spots when you use it up.

I like to buy big bags of whatever candy is my current "low medicine" and break them up into smaller ziplock bags. Or go nuts on the Halloween clearance candy, where you can get perfect mini–packs of Sour Patch Kids, Skittles, and Swedish Fish. I put those bags in a few places:

- Car
- Gym bag
- Purse
- Desk
- Nightstand
- Partner's nightstand

- Travel bag
- Winter jacket pocket
- Summer dog-walking bag
- Jogging fanny pack

Remember to choose foods that won't freeze or melt if you're putting them in your car!

When you're prepared to treat lows with "low medicine," it's a lot easier to stop yourself from grabbing 100 grams of carbs from the cupboard.

Remind yourself what happens when you binge

Still, tempted to binge? Be honest with yourself. When you binge during hypoglycemia, you are abusing your body with food. That might sound dramatic, but we both know your body is suffering from that binge after already suffering from the low blood sugar.

Talk yourself through the consequences of binge eating. Ask yourself a basic question: "Do I want to change this part of my life?"

If you're not willing to do the work — choosing the more challenging option instead of the easy one — then you'll keep getting the same results over and over.

During that urge to binge, ask yourself:

- How is bingeing during lows impacting your diabetes?
- How is it going to affect your energy the rest of the day?
- How is it affecting your weight?
- What's the aftermath? Is it worth it?
- How does it make you feel about yourself?
- Is it really worth it?

The more you can look honestly at the consequences of over-treating lows, the more you can remind yourself why you're going to manage this low differently.

Treating lows during exercise

Treating lows during exercise can be tricky because there are so many variables to consider.

- What's causing the low — how much extra insulin is causing the low?
- Do you need 5 grams, 15 grams, or 50 grams based on the cause of the low?
- How many carbs do you need if you plan to finish your workout?
- Or is your blood sugar dropping so rapidly that you truly need to stop, eat more, and rest?
- Maybe you could treat the low, wait 15 minutes, then restart?

What we know for sure, though, is this:

- You should absolutely be prepared *always* with fast-acting carbs while exercising.
- You should *not* use this as an opportunity to go nuts and eat *all the carbs*.
- You should consider calling 911 or using emergency glucagon if the low is more than you can manage safely with food, if you're struggling to stay on your feet, OR if you're feeling like you might pass out.
- You should *stop* exercising when you're low and treat the low thoughtfully.
- You should choose fat-free/fast-acting carbs to treat lows while exercising.
- You should give yourself at least 10-15 minutes for your blood sugar to rise before restarting.
- You should consider how much insulin is still active in your system before restarting.
- If you intend to continue exercising eventually, you might find it helpful to eat a more substantial carb source *after* the fast-acting carbs — like a small yogurt or a granola bar — to slowly soak up the extra IOB.

The more consistent and thoughtful you are in how you manage lows during exercise, the more likely you'll recover smoothly

without a dramatic rebound — and eventually continue exercising!
(More on exercise in the next chapter!)

If you do overeat during your next low
Yup, it's gonna happen. Even with all your guidelines in place and
new habits reinforced, it's still gonna happen again at some point
for three simple reasons:

- **You are human.** You're gonna overtreat the occasional low
  despite your best intention — especially if it's one of those
  lows that has you sweating and spinning and worrying about
  potential death. You're trying to save yourself.
- **You realize you overdosed on your insulin** or forgot to eat or
  something else that created the potential for a very intense low
  blood sugar. Overeating is a lifesaving risk you just might
  have to take.
- **Low blood sugars are really scary.** When you see those down
  arrows, you panic. Some lows are scarier than others. Some
  arrows are scarier than others depending on the circumstances.
  It's okay.

If you find yourself giving in to the urge to binge or possibly even
needing to binge out of severe panic and an effort to stay alive,
keep these things in mind:

- **If you're bingeing and you know you don't need 100+ grams
  of carbs for this low,** consider taking a very thoughtful dose
  of rapid-acting insulin to cover some of those carbs. Not all
  the carbs. Maybe not even half the carbs. Just cover some of
  those carbs with a teeny bit of insulin. Yes, you might still
  find yourself a bit high later on, but the first goal is to
  prevent another low blood sugar. Talk yourself through that
  urge to rage-bolus. Resist it. Take a very thoughtful dose to
  cover some of those extra carbs.
- **If you are seriously worried about your ability to survive
  this low blood sugar,** and that's your reason for bingeing,
  consider a few things: 1. Tell a friend/partner/family
  member. 2. Grab your emergency glucagon. 3. Consider calling

911. (Don't have emergency glucagon? Definitely read the next chapter in this book. Everyone who takes insulin should also be prescribed emergency glucagon!)

- **Just try to stay off the roller coaster.** If you do binge, the next decision that creates that roller coaster is the rage bolus. That's your opportunity to intervene. Take a deep breath. Take a teeny bit of insulin and simply accept that your time-in-range isn't going to be awesome for the rest of the day. Spending the day a little high is significantly better for your health than riding an exhausting, dangerous roller coaster. Just let the food and the insulin settle. Stay off the coaster.

Beyond the low: when you do need more...

Even if the low itself doesn't need more than 15 grams of carbs to get you back into a safe range, there are definitely lows that require a real serving of carbohydrates — with a careful dose of insulin.

Okay, so your liver contains backup glucose. It's like a storage unit of glucose to use between meals, while you're sleeping, and when you're low. If you have diabetes and you're taking insulin every day, your liver can't really save you from a low like it should in a non-diabetic. But your body still uses some of that stored glucose when you're low.

Now, if you've had a bunch of lows in the past few days (from an ongoing rollercoaster), then your liver's storage of backup glucose gets used up.

This can mean that eating 15 grams of thoughtful carbohydrates might bring your blood sugar back up, but your entire body still feels so drained and so weak.

Okay, that's when you might need a more legit serving of carbohydrates.

Ideally, it's not three bowls of ice cream. Instead, maybe it's a banana and peanut butter, or two slices of whole grain toast with butter, or a small bowl of oatmeal, or an apple with some cheese.

The point is: yes, you might need extra carbs sometimes, but you can still do this thoughtfully and carefully. Easier said than done! I know. But if you give yourself permission to eat a small meal of wholesome food, you don't have to binge. You can take a very careful dose of insulin to go with that meal.

Then take a deep breath, go distract yourself, and let your body recover.

Okay, six phrases to keep in your head

Get in the habit of reaching for these guidelines when you're dealing with your next low blood sugar.

- I will not overeat during hypoglycemia.
- I will choose my "low medicine" foods to treat low blood sugars.
- I will eat 8 to 15 grams of carbohydrates, depending on the circumstances.
- I will wait 15 minutes and distract myself with a glass of water, baby carrots, chewing gum, music, or being very patient.
- I am in control of how much food I eat during this low blood sugar.
- I care about my body. I will treat this low thoughtfully.

Ginger's example:

Well, I'll be honest: I can't eat glucose tabs much these days. I had a really bad experience with Norovirus when I was eight months pregnant. I had a ton of insulin on board. I was puking like crazy.

I couldn't keep anything down, even juice, not even a single sip of water. While my then-husband drove me to the hospital, I tried to eat glucose tabs. I couldn't keep them down. Five seconds of trying to eat a glucose tab resulted in more puking. That's when you know there's a problem!

Long story short: that's why I don't currently use the absolute best thing for low blood sugars. I associate them with Norovirus. It was brutal.

Okay, so that's my very graphic explanation of why I don't use glucose tabs very often these days.

Instead, I use specific things I can measure, like jelly beans, Sour Patch Kids, candy corn, and gummy Life-Savers. I can easily choose to just eat three or four. (If it's candy corn, I swear just three could bring you up 100 points. Be careful!)

I truly try to consume as little during a low blood sugar as possible.

I woke up the other morning at 5 a.m. at 50 mg/dL. I wanted to eat everything, but I also didn't want to ruin the entire rest of my day. Sounds dramatic, but we know it's possible! I truly wanted to eat four bowls of cereal. My brain was like, "Ooohhh, that would feel so good!"

Instead, I ate four Mike n' Ike candies. Then I made a cup of black coffee and watched movie trailers on YouTube. I wasn't thinking about cereal anymore. After 15 minutes of movie trailers, my blood sugar had risen just enough. More importantly, my brain felt better.

I am certain that following these guidelines for managing low blood sugar has helped me avoid diabetes-related weight gain and stay within my target range more easily. It also just keeps my energy levels high! I don't have time to waste feeling exhausted from the blood sugar roller coaster. I've got two kids. Tons of work. Dogs to walk! Weights to lift. Jogs to run. I need my energy! I am not going to let hypoglycemia steal my energy.

Hey, be nice to your body!

Yes, time-in-range, A1c, and joy can all benefit from your ability to follow thoughtful guidelines when treating lows.

When you learn how to treat lows thoughtfully, you set yourself up for success later in the day. Instead of a roller coaster, you might find yourself at 128 mg/dL. Sitting comfortably and safely in your target range.

You can't change the fact that diabetes happened to you, but you can change how much you let it ruin your day. When you choose to be in charge of how much food you eat during a low, you're choosing to have a better day. You're choosing to show diabetes who's boss! YOU!

You're also choosing to treat your body well.

Yes, there will still be days when you get stuck on that coaster, but the real goal is to treat your body well. To avoid abusing it with more food, more insulin, more lows, more highs.

When you find your brain begging you to eat everything in the cupboard, ask yourself, "What is the kindest thing I could do for my body right now?"

Chapter 6

LET'S LOOK AT THOSE FREQUENT LOWS

We all have lows. However, if you're experiencing low blood sugars every single day, this means your insulin doses need some fine-tuning. It's all about patterns!

Nothing will go as planned if you are getting too much or too little insulin. For example, just the tiniest bit too much basal/background insulin can cause dramatic low blood sugars while vacuuming the house, even when you don't have mealtime insulin on board.

On the other side, if you aren't getting enough basal/background insulin, you might find yourself constantly taking correction doses of rapid-acting insulin. That overlapping mess can lead to dramatic lows! You might actually need more basal/background insulin to prevent low blood sugars because this means you'll be taking less rapid-acting correction insulin.

Fine-tuning your insulin doses is complicated, because our insulin needs are truly different every day. But one thing you need to know for sure: frequent lows (or frequent highs) mean you are not getting the right amount of insulin.

Your insulin needs can change significantly throughout your life. What about the doses your doctor establishes when you first start taking insulin? Those are just estimates based on your weight and age! These doses need to be adjusted constantly — with support from your healthcare team as needed.

Tiny adjustments by just a few units or 5-10% of your total basal dose can have a huge impact on your ability to stay in your goal range whether you're sleeping, working, or jogging.

Ginger's example:

Even with 10 units as my current basal insulin dosage, I still adjust my dose up or down by 5-10% at times based on variables like my menstrual cycle, slight weight gain, really indulgent meals (pizza, cake, etc.), sudden stressful moments (like adopting a new dog), or the night before Thanksgiving day.

Over the course of years, my background insulin dose has changed a lot as my lifestyle habits, age, and body composition changed, too. Here's a look at my background insulin dose over the last 15 years:

- **At 20 years old — 32 units total basal insulin:** I was very sedentary, 150 lbs., with poor nutrition habits, and regularly overeating.
- **At 22 years old — 18 units total basal insulin:** I was very active teaching yoga, competing in powerlifting, at 155 lbs. but I had become very muscular. I was winning powerlifting competitions and following a structured moderate-carb diet.
- **At 28 years old — 17 units total basal insulin:** I was preparing for pregnancy, at 128 lbs., being thoughtful whole-food diet including some carbs and dessert, etc. I was very active with low-impact cardio (a lot of dog walks), and no longer doing heavy weightlifting.
- **At 30 years old — 11 units total basal insulin:** I was very active with daily cardio exercise and light weightlifting, at 125 pounds. As a busy mother of two, I was eating a flexible diet with plenty of whole foods and regular carbs.
- **At 32 years old — increased from 11 units to 16 units total basal insulin nearly overnight:** I was very active with daily cardio and light weights, at 120 lbs., but highly stressed for several months while managing the process of divorce with two small children. It was go go go.
- **At 36 years old — 10 units total basal insulin:** I was very active (mostly jogging or jumping rope and dog walks), at 122 lbs., eating a whole-foods diet with some carbs and room for a little bit of daily dessert.
- **Weird transition year:** I was experiencing tedious insulin resistance that didn't make sense based on my consistent

lifestyle habits. I talked to my endocrinologist about this and discovered many type Is are taking a GLP-I medication like Ozempic or Trulicity to manage insulin resistance.

- **At 37 years old — 9 units total basal insulin:** 115 lbs. I'm doing exactly the same as my 122 lbs. habits, but I started taking metformin and semaglutide (Ozempic). I initially lost more weight than I needed, but eventually, a reasonable appetite returned, and I could regain the weight I didn't intend to lose. Of course, my new insurance wouldn't cover it, so I gradually weened myself off of it.
- **At 38 years old — 10 to 11 units total basal insulin:** 120 lbs. I'm consistently managing this weight, and my body seems happy here. My insulin sensitivity is consistent. I decrease to 10 units if I start trending lower. I raise it to 11 units if it looks like I'm trending higher. This tiny adjustment makes all the difference.

Can you imagine if I'd kept the same background insulin dose over all these years? The big changes in doses came gradually as my body changed from a sedentary body to a powerlifter body to a light weights/cardio exercise body. If I hadn't made these changes, I'd probably be struggling with extreme blood sugar fluctuations and quite miserable!

Little adjustments are critical

Whether you use a pump or take insulin via injections/inhalations, little adjustments in your insulin doses are extremely important. The smallest changes in life can require changes in your basal/background insulin needs.

Changes like:

- Losing or gaining even just 5 pounds
- Starting a new habit of walking every day after lunch
- Joining a gym and lifting weights 3 days a week
- Reducing your alcohol consumption
- Starting a new medication
- Quitting smoking
- Going through a divorce
- Starting a new job

- Losing a loved one
- Menstrual cycle starting/ending
- Ovulation, menopause, pregnancy, etc.
- Puberty
- Transitioning to college life
- End of school transition to summer
- Back to school
- Holidays and food-focused celebrations
- Yada, yada, yada!

The list goes on and on.

You may only need an increased/decreased dose for a few days or a few weeks! But that tiny adjustment can make life so much easier when your sanity and overall health rely heavily on your ability to manage your blood sugar all day long. Learning how to make these tiny adjustments yourself at home is pretty critical.

You cannot wait three or six months before your next appointment. Reach out and get support from your healthcare team, but in the meantime, they should also be teaching you how to make adjustments on your own.

Don't settle for daily low blood sugars

You should not have to endure daily bouts of dramatic low blood sugars just because you have diabetes. Your insulin doses need to be adjusted!

I've heard from so many people over the years that they're experiencing frequent dramatic swings in their blood sugar levels.

One gal had called 911 three times in six months due to sudden severe hypoglycemia — and her doctor *didn't* adjust her background insulin.

This young woman was taking 30 units of long-acting insulin every night when she eventually determined that she only needed 20 units. She was taking 10 units *too* much because that was her doctor's initial estimate.

A 40-year-old man told me he was experiencing intense shaking, sweating, and hunger about an hour or two after eating. He was taking insulin with his meals, but he was taking way too much — per his doctor's instructions. No one taught him about hypoglycemia. He had type 2 diabetes, and it was assumed he was his insulin resistance and high blood sugar levels would prevent him from ever going low. He was experiencing severe hypoglycemia every single day after eating lunch.

Another woman who reached out to me was in her 60s and very active, but her new endocrinologist had suddenly told her to increase her long-acting insulin dose by 10 units. She followed his instructions and was experiencing scary hypoglycemia every afternoon during her routine 6-mile walk.

Guzzling juice and candy, trying to save her own life was exhausting. Eventually, she reduced her basal dose back down and was able to enjoy those long walks again. (And yes, she got a new endocrinologist, too.)

These are dramatic examples of getting too much insulin, but even a few units more than you need can wreak havoc on your daily life with diabetes. That is the power of insulin!

Is it your basal or your bolus insulin?

Pinpointing the cause of your lows (basal vs. bolus) is the trickiest part.

You're probably **getting too much basal/background** insulin if you:

- ...go low during a 1-mile walk without any rapid-acting insulin-on-board.
- ...go low during 30 minutes of weightlifting without any rapid-acting insulin-on-board.
- ...go low every single day despite careful meal dosing and you can't figure out why.
- ...feel like anything and everything can cause you to go low.

You probably **need more basal** insulin if you:

- ...are usually high three to four hours after eating.
- ...often can't correct a high blood sugar within four hours.
- ...generally feel like your mealtime/correction insulin "isn't working."

You're probably **getting too much mealtime/bolus** insulin if you:

- ...go low within three hours after eating, taking insulin with that meal.
- ...have to eat to keep your blood sugar from dropping ("feeding" your insulin).
- ...feel like anything and everything can cause you to go low.

You probably **need more mealtime/bolus** insulin if you:

- ...are usually high within two to three hours after eating.

First, you get your basal/background insulin dose established. That's the foundation of your house. Then, you start tweaking your mealtime/bolus insulin dose as needed.

Exercising without lows

Well, this is going to be an extremely condensed version of my book, *"Exercise with Type 1 Diabetes"* — which teaches you how to prevent highs and lows during any type of exercise.

But here are the most important nuggets you need to know:

- **Aerobic (cardio) exercise usually causes blood sugar to drop.** This includes jogging, walking, skating, vacuuming, gardening, cycling, swimming, jazzercise, etc. Anything where you are performing the same task for an extended period, like 10 minutes or longer. Glucose is your primary source of fuel during this type of exercise. You'll usually find that you need a significant reduction in your pump's basal rates or you need extra carbs (without extra insulin) to get through this type of exercise without dropping. But wait, more on this in a minute.

- **Anaerobic exercise usually causes blood sugar to rise.** This includes weightlifting, sprinting, intense spinning intervals, boxing, sparring, etc. Anything super intense for a minute or two then requires to pause, then repeat. This causes your body to convert lactic acid into glucose for fuel, and your liver can release stored glucose, too. You might find you actually need a small bolus of insulin before, during, or immediately after this type of exercise.

Insulin-on-board

Any type of exercise can cause your blood sugar to drop if you have too much insulin-on-board. Keep in mind that rapid-acting insulin (like Novolog, Humalog, Fiasp, etc.) stays in your system for about 4 to 5 hours. Inhaled insulin (Afrezza) stays in your system for about 60-90 minutes for smaller doses, and up to 3 hours for larger doses.

Exercising without lows starts with managing insulin-on-board before and during your workout.

- **If you take multiple daily injections:** This starts with getting your long-acting insulin dose as low as possible so you don't drop during exercise when you have no rapid-acting insulin on board. If your blood sugar drops when you only have long-acting insulin in your system, you are clearly getting too much long-acting insulin. After reducing your long-acting dose, you may find you need more rapid-acting insulin with meals. That's okay! That gives you more flexibility. You shouldn't have to feed your long-acting insulin with extra food.
- **If you use an insulin pump:** You'll need to experiment with temp-basal-rates or "activity mode" starting about an hour before your exercise. For example, you might find you need to reduce your basal rate by 75 percent depending on the duration and intensity of your workout. Milder exercise might only call for a reduction of 25 to 50 percent.

You've gotta take good notes! Create your own experiments by performing the same type of exercise at the same time of day.

Making small adjustments in the experiment until you can safely predict and prevent lows or highs.

Exercising in a "fasted state" is easiest

When you exercise *before* eating, you immediately reduce your risk of going low because you don't have that big ol' bolus of rapid-acting insulin on board.

Your risk of going low during exercise is significantly lower if it's been...

- **3 to 4 hours since your last dose of rapid-acting liquid insulin.**
    - **Injected or pumped insulin:** If you take a bolus of rapid-acting insulin (Novolog, Humalog, Fiasp, etc.) via injection or pump, that insulin is most active in your bloodstream for about 3 to 4 hours. If you exercise during that 4-hour window, your risk of going low is significantly likely. If you can time your workout to take place after that 3 to 4-hour window, you can hugely reduce your risk of hypoglycemia.
    - **If you use an insulin pump:** You will likely need to reduce your basal rates significantly before aerobic exercise to prevent hypoglycemia. We'll discuss this in great detail later.
- **60 to 90 minutes since your last dose of ultra-rapid inhaled insulin.**
    - **Inhaled insulin:** If you use inhaled insulin for your meals or corrections, that insulin is most active in your bloodstream for 60 to 90 minutes. Exercising during that time frame increases your risk of going low.

Why? Because the less rapid-acting insulin you have active in your bloodstream, the less glucose is going to be rapidly used for fuel.

When you don't have a big bolus of insulin-on-board to grab glucose easily for fuel, your muscles use less glucose and burn more fat for fuel.

Ginger's example:

These days, I start my mornings with a 45-minute dog walk, followed eventually by a 30-minute jog. I perform all of this in a "fasted state" which means I haven't eaten food. This means I also haven't taken any rapid-acting insulin for meals in at least 4 hours.

I can wake up at 80 mg/dL and exercise for over an hour without going low because I don't have a bolus of rapid-acting insulin on board.

- **If I wake up a little high,** I take a teeny smidge of insulin to start the correction while letting the exercise bring it down the rest of the way.
- **If I wake up low,** I eat as few carbohydrates as possible to treat the low, then continue with my workout plans when it feels safe.

I can create this exact same fasted environment for my afternoon dog walk by eating lunch after the dog walk instead of before. For an evening workout, I'd eat my dinner after the workout, too.

Fasted exercise isn't the only way. But it can create a much smoother, safer, and simpler approach to exercising without highs and lows.

Fine-tuning with small, careful adjustments

When making adjustments in your basal/background insulin dose(s), it's important to start small. Never make an adjustment of more than 1 to 3 units at a time. If you're more sensitive to insulin, a 1-unit increase/decrease is plenty. If you're more resistant, a 3-unit increase/decrease may be more appropriate.

Then, let that new dose prove itself for two to three days before making any further decisions — unless it is glaringly obvious that it is too much or too little.

The bigger message is: don't be afraid to make small, thoughtful adjustments to your background insulin. Small and thoughtful adjustments. You cannot wait for your next appointment six months to make those tweaks. It's just too long to wait.

And actually, it's dangerous to wait. If you're not getting the right amount of insulin, your health is suffering. And there are just too many reasons your body needs small adjustments to your insulin doses all the time.

Taking insulin means paying very close attention to the patterns in your blood sugar. If you're going low every single day, something ain't right! Don't suffer. Take action. Make adjustments.

Chapter 7

HEY, YOU SHOULD KNOW ABOUT GLUCAGON

There's a whole chapter on this because too many people still know about today's single-step emergency glucagon options! Many doctors are either still prescribing the very outdated and complicated red glucagon kit that nobody wants to use, or they aren't prescribing emergency glucagon at all.

If you take insulin, you should have emergency glucagon in your kitchen, at work, and next to your bed.

First, what is glucagon?

Okay, glucagon is a hormone that tells your liver to release stored sugar, also known as glycogen. Every human body produces glucagon — some better than others!

- Glucagon: a natural human hormone
- Glycogen: stored sugar in your liver

In people without diabetes, glucagon naturally prevents low blood sugars — like while you're sleeping or if you skip breakfast. Glucagon tells your liver to release that stored sugar, use it for energy, and keep your blood sugar steady.

Glucagon is kind of like the diabetes version of an "Epi-pen" for peanut allergies. It's a rapid single dose of medication that is designed to prevent disaster and save your life.

In people with diabetes taking insulin, this whole glucagon function is all screwed up. Your body isn't naturally regulating this in response to the insulin you're taking via injection or pump. Thus, all the tedious, exhausting, and sometimes very scary low blood sugars!

Emergency glucagon medications were originally meant to be used on you by another person when you were struggling to function or unconscious due to severe hypoglycemia. Today's glucagon options, though, are so easy to use that many people give themselves glucagon during severe hypoglycemia before they've lost consciousness.

Today's emergency glucagon options

The following are today's available glucagon options as of April 2024.

These medications are intended to be very easy for friends or family members to administer to a person living with diabetes experiencing severe hypoglycemia. Many people with diabetes have reported giving themselves emergency glucagon during moderate-to-severe low blood sugars.

- **Nasal glucagon (Baqsimi):** This glucagon is administered through the nose. It's a very compact container with an obvious "spout" that sits inside the nostril. Two spots for your fingers allow you to pull down and administer the glucagon spray directly into the nose.
- **Glucagon pen (Gvoke HypoPen):** This is very similar to the Epi-Pen, designed like a thick pen. You simply remove the cap and press the tip of the HypoPen against the thigh. It auto-injects liquid glucagon.
- **Glucagon prefilled syringe (Gvoke PFS):** This is the same premixed liquid glucagon but in a syringe that requires you to manually inject the syringe into the thigh muscle.
- **Glucagon vial & syringe (Gvoke Kit):** This requires an additional step of drawing the premixed glucagon liquid into the syringe and then injecting it into the thigh. This is a premixed glucagon in a vial that comes with a syringe, allowing you to draw up the dose manually and inject it directly into the thigh muscle.
- **Glucagon pen (Zegalogue):** This is very similar to the Epi-Pen, designed like a thick pen. You simply remove the cap and press the tip of the HypoPen against the thigh muscle. It auto-injects liquid glucagon.

liquid glucagon.

- **Glucagon prefilled syringe (Zegalogue PFS):** This is the same premixed liquid glucagon but in a syringe that requires you to manually inject the syringe into the thigh muscle.

Generally speaking, injected glucagon has little-to-no side effects beyond a rise in blood sugar. You may notice somewhat resistant blood sugar levels during the following 24 hours simply because that hormone is still present, telling your liver to release stored glucose. This usually settles down within 24 hours.

Some people have reported vomiting and intense headaches after administering glucagon. Others have little-to-no side effects. Your post-glucagon experience can vary depending on the circumstances and your body's reactions to different types of glucagon.

When should you use emergency glucagon?

While most lows can be treated with carbs, emergency glucagon is meant for those lows when eating or drinking isn't an option.

Here are a few of the scenarios when you or someone else might administer glucagon:

- If you've significantly overdosed on insulin or took the wrong type of insulin.
- If food or drink isn't correcting your blood sugar.
- If you are unable to physically eat or drink.
- If you have a stomach virus and vomit repeatedly, unable to keep food down.
- If you feel like you might pass out and fear food won't be enough to save you.
- If you are seizing, unconscious, or unresponsive.

Glucagon & alcohol

When you have significant amounts of alcohol in your bloodstream, glucagon will not be as effective. This is because alcohol suppresses liver glucose production while your liver is focused on processing the alcohol you've consumed.

Teach your friends & family how to use it

While we all hope it never happens, your friends or family might have to use glucagon on you someday. But that's only gonna happen if they actually know where you've stored your glucagon and how to use it!

Teach your friends, family members, and coworkers about emergency glucagon. Teach them where you store it, how to use it, and when to use it. You should also tell them, "But first, call 911. If you're not comfortable administering glucagon, call 911. If you think I'm struggling with severe hypoglycemia, call 911. Just call 911."

Hopefully, they never actually have to do any of the above. At the very least, you will have taught them when to call 911.

Ginger's example:

So, I mentioned a few chapters ago my bout with Norovirus when I was eight months pregnant. Yeah, that was brutal — and I did *not* have emergency glucagon. I had 10 units of insulin on board and just puked up all the food those 10 units covered. I couldn't keep juice or glucose tabs down.

My blood sugar was around 40 mg/dL and continuing to drop.

Now, this was before today's single-step glucagon options existed, but even an old-school emergency glucagon kit would've completely changed this experience. I would've still needed to go to the hospital — because of the severe dehydration that comes with repeated vomiting — but I could've treated the super scary hypoglycemia with glucagon if I had filled the prescription. Our drive to the hospital would've been much calmer. The immediate life-threatening urgency would've been taken care of by the glucagon.

More recently, I accidentally took twice as much insulin as I needed for the last meal I ate before bed. I didn't realize my mistake until I woke up around 2 a.m., and the room was spinning.

I mean, the room was truly spinning. My feet felt like they weren't really on the floor. Like I was floating or walking on waves? It wasn't fun. I experienced a few dramatic lows in my early 20s before CGMs existed, but this was intense.

I got myself downstairs to the kitchen. I could still eat, but food didn't feel like it was going to be enough. I ate one bowl of cereal and gave myself a Gvoke prefilled syringe of glucagon.

I knew it was probably more than I needed, but I didn't care. The only way I was going to feel safe falling asleep again was with glucagon. I knew the power of this hormone would keep me alive. I knew I didn't need to panic because I had glucagon in my system. I knew I was going to be okay. (And I was.)

Get some glucagon before you wish you had it

If you have it on hand and you're experiencing a bad low, glucagon can also prevent all that binge-eating. It's about safety. It's about staying alive and knowing you're going to be okay.

You might think you don't need glucagon if you "feel your lows" or have never passed out from hypoglycemia, but today's glucagon is so easy to use that it's worth getting some. There can be a lot of shame and embarrassment that comes with using or needing glucagon, but there shouldn't be.

Insulin is no joke — you are taking injections every day of a medication that can kill you!

Emergency glucagon is a must-have. It only takes one bout of Norovirus or taking 10 units of the wrong insulin to wish you had it. Just get some.

Chapter 8

Insulin is one of the most complicated medications on the planet. A smidge too much can nearly kill you. Not enough insulin tears down your body over time — quickly or slowly, depending on which type of diabetes you live with.

It's exhausting. And yet, here you are, dealing with it every single day. Showing up is the first step. The next step is owning your attitude — your mindset — and putting as much joy into your life as possible.

Your mindset matters

Thriving with any type of diabetes starts with how you look at it. If you roll your eyes at this, then you really, really need to hear it again. Your attitude and mindset determine everything, actually.

For example, the following is true about everyone with diabetes at some moment:
- You will experience high blood sugars.
- You will experience low blood sugars.
- You will miscalculate your insulin doses.
- You will go low during exercise.
- You will go high when you least expect it.
- Diabetes will interrupt something really important.
- Diabetes will cost you money.
- Diabetes will cause you at least a bit of stress, frustration, and anxiety.

But your mindset, attitude, and perception of diabetes truly determine the following:
- You will be angry every week because of diabetes.
- You will feel sorry for yourself because of diabetes.

- You will feel resentful towards people without diabetes.
- You will feel depressed and unlucky because of diabetes.
- Diabetes will get in the way of your goals.
- Diabetes will make it harder for you to feel joy.
- Diabetes will hold you back.

Your mindset, attitude, and perception of diabetes can also determine this:

- Diabetes will fill you with gratitude because you can keep living.
- Diabetes will fill you with pride in what you face every day.
- Diabetes will give you motivation to be diligent about your habits.
- Diabetes will teach you more about nutrition than most will ever learn.
- Diabetes will make you feel remarkably resilient.
- Diabetes will make you feel grateful to be still alive.

What does all of this have to do with low blood sugars?

It's your mindset. Either you're a victim of low blood sugars or you're a survivor. Either your low blood sugars are in charge of you, or you're in charge of them. The low blood sugar tells you what to eat, or you manage that low blood sugar like you're in charge! (Because you *are* in charge!)

If you want this part of your life to be different, make it different. It's truly that simple. But it starts with simply owning your attitude, your mindset, and then your actions. If you're going to eat the whole box of cereal, own it. Don't blame it on the low blood sugar and the insulin. Own it. You can't change it if you still believe it's something else's fault.

You are in charge. That doesn't mean you have to be perfect or know everything. It just means you take responsibility for your decisions and your actions. It means you're always open to learning and evolving. It means you treat yourself with kindness when you make mistakes. It means you try your best and move on quickly when you struggle. Then you try again.

You are in charge of *your* lows. You are in charge of your life living with type 1 or type 2 diabetes. Make it what you want it to be.

You are not alone

When most of the people around you seem to effortlessly produce exactly the right amount of insulin all day long, living with any type of diabetes can feel pretty darn lonely.

But you are not alone! I'm not going to report stats from the World Health Organization on how many millions of people live with type 1 and type 2 diabetes. You know there are millions. That doesn't change the day-to-day feeling of loneliness.

Creating in-person relationships with diabetes isn't easy. When you spot someone at the grocery store with an insulin pump, it would be awfully awkward to walk up and try to establish some sort of friendship. (Although, it does always feel good to see people with diabetes walking around "in the wild" just like you.)

Instead, this is one of the good things about social media: you can find genuine content created by real people with diabetes — and I guarantee it will help you feel less alone. You can also create friendships with people all across the globe who are in your shoes. It's actually pretty easy to get started.

Instagram: Start by searching a hashtag like #diabetes, #t2d, #type2diabetes, #type1diabetes, or #t1d. Without "following" anyone, you can simply find diabetes-related content to peruse with the search results. But you can also find very outgoing diabetes-related accounts. Follow them! Reach out and say hello. Look at who else follows them — you'll find a huge variety of people who talk about their diabetes nearly every day. That doesn't mean you have to, but simply following their content can help you feel less alone.

Facebook: This is a great place to find chat groups. If you search specifics like "women with diabetes," "inhaled insulin," or "parents of children with diabetes," you will find a variety of groups. Request to join. Get a feel for the vibe of that group. If it's not a good fit, find another one.

Twitter…I mean, "X": Like Instagram, you can find a wide variety of people and content talking all about any type of diabetes. Twitter also includes occasional live chats hosted by different accounts. Start with #t1d, #type1diabetes, #GBdoc, #diabetes, #t2d, #diabeteschat, and #diabetes.

YouTube & Podcasts: There are some really wonderful YouTube channels hosted by real people with diabetes that focus on different aspects of diabetes, like technology, nutrition, everything, and more! Many podcasts also feature their episodes on YouTube. Start with: @DiabetesNerd, @DiabetesStrong, @TypeOneTalks, @Diabetech, @DiabeticsDoingThings, @RiselyHealth, @ScottJohnsonDiabetes, @YourDiabetesInsider, @TheHangryWoman, @TheLPodcast, and @HappyDiabeticTV.

HoneyHealth: This is a free app designed by people living with diabetes! It's filled with different groups hosted by a person with type 1 or type 2 diabetes, and regular new videos. You can also connect your CGM data to the app and get helpful reports on your time-in-range, patterns, and progress towards your goals. Find my group: Ginger's T1D Diary.

Thanks to social media, I've made lasting friendships with people all over the globe. It's impossible to put a price on the value of seeing other people face the same challenges you face. There's a lot of noise and nonsense on social media, but you can find the good stuff, too. I encourage you to give it a chance if you haven't already.

One more thing…

Low blood sugars are scary. You have every right to freak out, but it's worth digging into those other skills to manage your lows carefully. Making an effort to manage how much food you eat during a low can have a big impact on other parts of your life — starting with the pride you feel when you know you are in charge of your relationship with food and diabetes!

This affects every bit of your daily joy.

Do not let any type of this disease steal your joy. You are one very resilient human being. You are waking up every single day to deal with this disease again and again on top of the many other stressful parts of real life. You are resilient!

Low blood sugars are scary. Your body deserves to be treated well during those scary lows. This book, I hope, helps you treat your body with more kindly with food while feeling more pride in how you manage low blood sugars.

Words & Phrases You Need to Know

Here are a few words or phrases you need to know about diabetes management. Most of these words pop up frequently in this book.

- **Aerobic exercise:** Cardio exercise is a type of physical activity performed at an intensity you can sustain without stopping for an extended period of time.
- **Anaerobic exercise:** Commonly known as high-intensity exercises or strength training, a type of physical activity performed at an intensity that can only be performed in short bursts.
- **Bolus insulin:** A dose of rapid-acting insulin taken to cover meals or to correct high blood sugar.
- **Basal/background insulin:** Insulin that covers your background insulin needs is delivered via an insulin pump (with basal rates) or an injection of long-acting insulin.
- **Carbohydrates:** Carbohydrates are one of the three macronutrients carbohydrates, fat, and protein in the food you eat. While all three can affect blood sugar levels and insulin needs, carbohydrates usually have the most dramatic impact on blood sugar levels and require the most planning for insulin dosing and blood sugar management.
- **Closed-loop insulin pump:** Also referred to as "looping," closed-loop pumps are insulin pumps that communicate directly with your continuous glucose monitor (CGM) and automatically make adjustments in your insulin dosages to prevent fluctuations. Brand names include Omnipod 5, Tandem t:Slim, and Medtronic 670G and 770G.
- **Continuous glucose monitor (CGM):** Diabetes technology that measures blood sugar levels without pricking your finger. Brand names include Freestyle Libre, Dexcom, and Eversense. CGMs are highly recommended for anyone living with type I diabetes.
- **Correction dose:** The insulin you take to correct high blood sugar levels.

- **Diabetic ketoacidosis (DKA) / ketones:** This is a life-threatening condition caused by too little insulin and usually accompanied by very high blood sugars. While there are safe circumstances in which ketones are present (nutritional ketosis, for example), ketones caused by too little insulin in your body can lead to severe vomiting, dehydration, coma, and death. Talk to your healthcare team to get ketone strips for measuring ketone levels during high blood sugars, illness, etc.

- **Fasted exercise:** Exercising when you don't have a dose of insulin in your system for a meal.

- **Glucose:** The sugar in your bloodstream! This book uses "blood sugar" or "blood glucose" to imply the level on your CGM or glucose meter.

- **Glucagon:** A hormone produced by the pancreas that tells your liver to release stored glucose. In those without T1D, your body naturally produces glucagon between meals to prevent low blood sugar during exercise. In those of us with T1D, this natural regulation of glucagon is dysfunctional. Emergency glucagon kits contain a large dose of glucose to be administered during severe hypoglycemia. A large dose of glucagon tells your liver to release a large amount of stored glucose to restore your blood sugar back up to a safe level.

- **Goal range/target range:** Your personal blood sugar goals. The standard recommended target range by the American Diabetes Association is 80 to 180 mg/dL. The more you learn about blood sugar management, the tighter your target range might become. You may have a looser target range due to fear of hypoglycemia, inability to feel symptoms of hypoglycemia, your age, etc. That's okay! Your goal range should be thoughtfully decided with support from your healthcare team to help you be as safe and healthy as you can.

- **Hypoglycemia / Low blood sugar:** Blood sugar levels below 70 mg/dL. Throughout this book, I will refer to hypoglycemia as low blood sugar. *Severe low blood sugar* is generally considered anything below 55 mg/dL when your risk of losing consciousness or experiencing a seizure increases significantly.

- **Hyperglycemia / high blood sugar:** Also known as hyperglycemia, blood sugar levels above your goal range. For some, that's over 150 mg/dL; for others, it's over 225 mg/dL. Throughout this book, I will refer to hyperglycemia as high blood sugar, with a level of 180 mg/dL as the general standard. What qualifies as high blood sugar can vary greatly from person to person depending on your personal comfort levels, access to newer diabetes technology and medications, and goals. Exercising with blood sugar levels over 250 mg/dL can increase your risk of developing ketones — talk to your healthcare team about reasonable goals for you!

- **Insulin-on-board (IOB):** The insulin that is already active in your body. Mostly, IOB talks about rapid-acting insulin delivered via injection, pump, or inhalation. IOB includes both bolus and basal insulin.

- **Inhaled insulin:** One of the newer insulins on the market that delivers ultra-rapid-acting insulin via oral inhalation. For simplicity throughout this book, I will include inhaled insulin as part of rapid-acting insulin discussions. Brand names include Afrezza. Read more at GingerVieira.com/diabetes.

- **Insulin sensitivity/insulin resistance:** Your body's need for insulin can vary based on increasing insulin resistance (which means you need more insulin to manage in-range blood sugar levels) or increasing insulin sensitivity (which means you need less insulin to manage in-range blood sugar levels. Neither one is completely good or completely bad. Many natural factors can cause a body to become more insulin resistant — like growth hormones, reproductive hormones, excitement, stress, etc. Other factors are typically less desirable — like weight gain, lack of physical activity, a diet high in processed fatty foods, excessive stress, smoking cigarettes, drinking too much caffeine, and too little sleep. Increasing your insulin sensitivity is usually ideal because the less insulin you need to manage in-range blood sugar levels, the easier it will likely be. Factors that increase insulin sensitivity include weight loss, regular exercise, a cleaner diet, adequate sleep, limited caffeine, and manageable stress levels.

- **Intermittent fasting:** An approach to eating during certain times of day and not eating during others. The most popular is a 16:8 approach, which means you fast for 16 hours and eat your day's worth of calories within 8 hours. Many people approach this by eating their last meal before bed and not eating again until the next afternoon, around 1 or 2 p.m.

- **Long-acting insulin:** Insulin that is taken once or twice a day to serve your basal/background insulin needs. Every person with type 1 diabetes needs basal/background insulin of some kind at all times. Brand names include Lantus, Toujeo, Tresiba, Lyumjev, and Levemir.

- **Pancreas:** The organ responsible for producing insulin, amylin, glucagon, and much more! This is the organ that your immune system is attacking as a person with T1D. Technically, your pancreas is healthy, but your immune system is dysfunctional.

- **Rapid-acting insulin:** Insulin that begins working within an hour and stays in your system for anywhere from 3 to 6 hours. It can be used via a pump for both basal and bolus insulin doses. Can be used via pen or syringe for bolus insulin needs. Brand names include Novolog, Humalog, Fiasp, Apidra, Admelog, and Afrezza (inhaled, ultra-rapid).

- **Resilience:** You! You are the epitome of resilience. You get back up and try again over and over and over. You are resilient. You have resilience.

- **Type 1 diabetes:** A chronic illness defined by an autoimmune attack on the cells of your pancreas that produce insulin and several other critical hormones. T1D also includes latent autoimmune deficiency in adults (LADA) and can develop at any age. There are actually *six* hormones people with T1D don't produce properly. There is no cure at this time. Recent FDA approval of the drug teplizumab has been shown to delay the full onset of T1D if it's administered in the earliest stages of the disease.

- **Type 2 diabetes:** A metabolic disorder defined by insulin resistance and dysfunctional insulin production. People with T2D may struggle to produce normal amounts of insulin or properly use the insulin they do produce. Contrary to mainstream media, it is *not* caused by sugary diets or weight gain, but lifestyle habits can play a role in the development of the disease. A significant percentage of people with T2D *cannot* simply reverse the condition through diet and weight loss.

About the Author

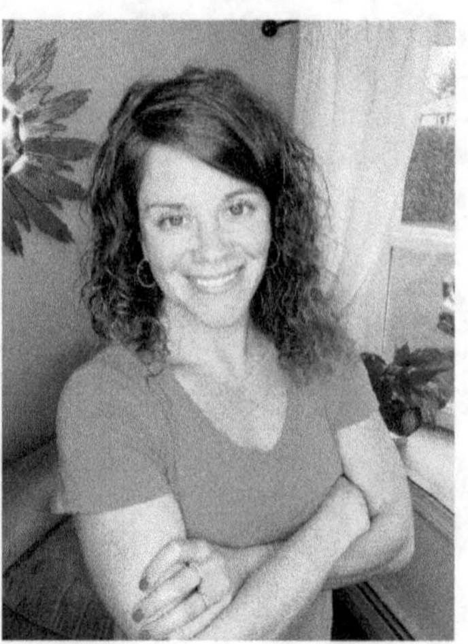

Ginger Vieira has lived with type 1 diabetes since 1999. She also lives with celiac disease, fibromyalgia, and POTS. She is thriving and loving life!

Once upon a time, Ginger was a personal trainer, yoga instructor, and competitive powerlifter. Today, she is an author, journalist, video creator, and health content specialist. She lives in Vermont with her beautiful kiddos, a handsome fella, and two dogs.

Find Ginger:

- GingerVieira.com
- YouTube.com/@DiabetesNerd
- Instagram.com/GingerVieira.t1d
- Linkedin.com/in/GingerVieira

Ginger's books:

- Stop Overeating During Low Blood Sugars with Diabetes
- Exercise with Type 1 Diabetes
- Dealing with Diabetes Burnout
- Pregnancy with Type 1 Diabetes
- Emotional Eating with Diabetes
- When I Go Low (for kids)
- Ain't Gonna Hide My T1D (for kids)

Love the book?

Leave a 5-star review on Amazon!